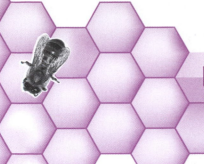

Foundations in Nursing and Health Care

Uncovering Skills for Practice

Carol Chapelhow
Sandra Crouch
Melanie Fisher
Anna Walsh
Series Editor: Lynne Wigens

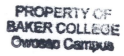

Published in 2005 by:
Nelson Thornes Ltd
Delta Place
27 Bath Road
CHELTENHAM
GL53 7TH
United Kingdom

05 06 07 08 09 / 10 9 8 7 6 5 4 3 2 1

A catalogue record for this book is available from the British Library

ISBN 0 7487 9261 9

Illustrations by Clinton Banbury
Page make-up by Florence Production Ltd

Printed in Great Britain by Ashford Colour Press

Contents

Acknowledgements

The authors would like to acknowledge the contribution that students, both past and present, and colleagues, both educational and clinical, have made to the development of this book. Much of this has been the driving force for our philosophy on clinical skill development.

We are also grateful to our husbands, families and friends, not only for their support and encouragement but also for their patience, tolerance and forbearance.

We would also like to thank the following people:

Dr Ann Smith for the use of the template she developed

Helen Smith for her inspiring and positive comments when she reviewed our initial draft

Alison Davidson both for listening and for encouraging us.

Introduction

If you are considering undertaking or are already engaged in education to qualify as a health care professional, this book has been written for you. Although our primary target is nursing students (and we refer throughout the text to the terms 'nurse' and 'nursing') the principles applied in this book can be transferred to a number of health care professionals who are learning to develop skills for caring.

We wrote this book because we saw that there was need for a text that helped students to learn 'how to learn' to become an expert nurse. In our experience many student nurses find clinical skill development difficult. One reason for this is that many clinical colleagues find it difficult to explain exactly what they do. This is because much of what they do is on an unconscious level (Benner 1984, Luker and Kenrick 1992, Meerabeau 1992, MacLeod 1996, Meyer and Batehup 1997). This book shares the way that many nurses view their work. Unlike the clinical skills books that have been published to date, our thoughts and ideas take a global perspective rather than purely focusing on the task. Many textbooks will provide you with a 'how to do it' menu, but this book goes an important step further by acknowledging the complexity of the care required. After all, to any nurse in today's clinical settings the task is a small part of any nursing intervention. In order to do this we tie motor skills in with psychological skills and the skills of critical thinking and making judgements. We introduce our template and model as tools to assist you on the way. Throughout the book we have acknowledged the uncertain nature of nurses' work.

We have used the term 'clinical skills' as an all-encompassing term for a variety of activities performed by a nurse. It brings to mind a series of tasks but we feel strongly that clinical skills are more than tasks. The components of skill delivery are 'unpacked', thus allowing you to examine your own knowledge requirements and deficits. This book offers a pathway of development to assist the novice learner to achieve skill acquisition and mastery. As learning is best achieved by continuous development we have taken a progressive approach to clinical skills. We take the reader on Benner's (1984) journey from novice to expert, culminating in the presentation of the Meaningful Assimilation of Skills for Care (MASC) model, which incorporates a template for all clinical skills. Central to our model is the belief that personal and professional knowledge underpins and shapes the type of practitioner that you become.

Succinctly describing what nurses do is difficult, as most nurses practise in a variety of different social contexts and with very unpredictable working days. They also have diverse values and beliefs – about themselves, society, health and nursing. Nursing has been traditionally seen as women's work (Gamarnikow 1978, 1991; Oakley 1984). Perhaps because of this, nursing hasn't developed a formal language to describe the work that nurses do. As a result there is no recognition of the complexity of many of the clinical skills that nurses perform in their daily work. However, if these skills were not performed in their complexity the patients and the National Health Service (NHS) would be left to pick up the pieces and the costs. The MASC model explores and clarifies the complexities that are inherent in today's health care arena.

Developing skills to meet the needs of patients in health care today is an onerous task. Educators and clinicians alike are under pressure to assist in the development of nurses who possess both the fundamental skills associated with the traditional role of the nurse and also more contemporary skills associated with government initiatives.

How to use this book

We'd like you to read this book from cover to cover; however, as ex-students and avid book users we know and understand that you will probably read the list of contents and the index and then dip in and out of chapters. While we have written the book to take you on a journey, we appreciate that, although many people prefer to start at the beginning and go straight to their destination, others will always take the scenic route. To those who do take the scenic route, all that we would ask is that you don't miss any of the 'scenery' of the book along the way. In keeping with the rest of the titles in the Foundations in Nursing and Health Care series we have incorporated activities that, if you complete them, will equip you for your journey.

The chapters have been written in a way that provides you with not only information but also reflective activities, case studies and exercises to enable you to examine your own practice. Each chapter outlines the learning outcomes and key words used.

In **Chapter 1** we examine the concept of clinical skills from our perspective: what are they, what do we mean by the term 'clinical skill' and what are the complexities and diversities of skill delivery. We examine the importance of integrating knowledge and understanding from a range of sources.

In **Chapter 2** we encourage students to think more laterally about skill development. We unpack the elements of skill delivery and provide students with ideas on how they might approach learning a skill based on 'essential' components. We explore some of these components such as: reflection, critical thinking, decision-making and acknowledge the influence of individual approaches to learning and knowledge acquisition. We suggest that students think of learning a skill as a complex process requiring a number of 'enabling' skills, rather than one single, discrete activity.

In **Chapter 3** we take the process of learning to become an expert nurse a step further and build on the essential components outlined in the previous chapter. We examine what we believe to be the fundamental or 'enabling skills' of nursing practice – assessment, communication, professional judgement and decision-making, record keeping and documentation, risk management and managing uncertainty. There are a number of exercises that are designed to enable you to begin acquiring these skills. Some of the exercises used are examples from your daily life whereas others are very much based in nursing practice. As this book is focused on taking you on the journey that will help you in your clinical skill development it means that this is a very long chapter.

In **Chapter 4** we introduce you to our template and model. We select a number of scenarios from practice and apply the model and template to illustrate how skill development can be adjusted to accommodate the uniqueness of each clinical encounter. By examining some of the more 'complex' skills, we not only demonstrate the flexibility of the template and model but also explore the impact of wider issues in health, such as legislation and policy. We examine a variety of clinical situations and step by step begin to fit the pieces of the jigsaw together.

In **Chapter 5** we explore both the importance of multidisciplinary working and how you can begin to acquire the skills that will help you to make an effective contribution to a multidisciplinary team. Health professionals have a variety of complementary skills and in this chapter we examine how these can be best used to enable effective and efficient patient care in today's NHS.

Chapter 6 is our final chapter, in which we examine the development of skills for caring in a much wider context. The skills you need to acquire and master throughout the course of your career will be dictated by service users and reinforced by government policy. The key principles of the MASC model can be applied to assist you in lifelong learning and in this chapter we explore some of the underpinning 'drivers' that will determine what some of those skills may be.

Traditionally, clinical skills have been taught as isolated tasks or procedures. Consequently many of today's clinical skills textbooks have been developed from procedure manuals. Unfortunately this approach to skills development is limited. While this approach is useful when learning less complex psychomotor skills such as floristry or interior design it has limited use in nursing, as this is a complex and dynamic subject that utilises what Tichen and Ersser (2001) call 'professional craft knowledge'.

We hope you enjoy reading this book and wish you luck on your exciting journey from 'novice' to' expert'.

References

Benner, P. (1984) *From Novice to Expert: Excellence and power in clinical nursing practice*. Addison Wesley, Menlo-Park, CA.

Gamarnikow, E. (1978) Sexual division of labour: the case of nursing. In: Kuhn, A. and Wolpe, A.M. (eds) *Feminism and Materialism: Women and modes of production*. Routledge & Kegan Paul, London.

Gamarnikow, E. (1991) Nurse or woman: gender or professionalism in reformed nursing 1860–1923. In: Holden, P. and Littlewood, J. (eds) *Anthropology and Nursing*. Routledge, London.

Luker, K. and Kenrick, M. (1992) An explanatory study of the sources of influence on the clinical decisions of community nurses. *Journal of Advanced Nursing*, **17**, 457–466.

MacLeod, M. (1996) *Practising Nursing – Becoming Experienced*. Churchill Livingstone, Edinburgh.

Meerabeau, L. (1992) Tacit knowledge; an untapped resource or a methodological headache? *Journal of Advanced Nursing*, **17**, 1108–1112.

Meyer, J. and Batehup, L. (1997) Action research in health care practice: nature, present concerns and future possibilities. *Nursing Times Research*, **2**, 3175–3186.

Oakley, A. (1984) The importance of being a nurse. *Nursing Times*, **80**(50), 24–27.

Tichen, A. and Ersser, S.J. (2001) The nature of professional craft knowledge. In: Higgs, J. and Tichen, A. (eds) *Practice Knowledge and Expertise in the Health Professions*. Butterworth-Heinemann, Oxford.

1

Our philosophy

Learning outcomes

By the end of this chapter you should be able to:

- Explain what is meant by the term 'clinical skill'
- Identify the key skills inherent in delivering care
- Discuss the importance of integrating knowledge and understanding from a range of sources when learning 'skills for practice'.

Keywords

Holistic care

Care that considers more than just the physical needs of patients. By looking at all the patient's needs, particularly the emotional and social needs, and how they interrelate, the care is enhanced and individualised. Over 2000 years ago, Hippocrates suggested, 'It is more important to know what sort of a person has a disease than to know what sort of a disease a person has.'

Background

Do you remember what it was that made you want to be a nurse? Did you have a mental picture of 'doing things' for people who are ill? When we have asked students at interview what they think nurses working with adult patients do, they readily suggest things such as giving out medicines and recording observations. These activities are easy to identify and are often referred to as practical or clinical skills. Sometimes the students also identify listening to, and educating, patients. All these are very important aspects of nursing care but if we think about care in terms of discrete 'activities' such as these we are guilty of breaking down care into a series of tasks. In reality the qualified nurse carries out all these 'tasks' at the same time, appearing to do it effortlessly and, having completed the care, manages also to have learned a lot about the patient.

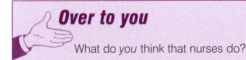

Over to you

What do *you* think that nurses do?

Learning practical/clinical skills is a fundamental part of learning to be a nurse. However, in order to become skilled practitioners we need to be able to put all aspects of care together to provide **holistic care**, which is sensitive to all the patient's needs. Therefore the 'tasks' that we perform need to be tailored to the needs of the individual.

For example, one patient we are administering medicines to might be feeling sick, refuse to take them or want to know all about them before they take them, whereas another patient may just swallow the medicines without even being asked to. Therefore the patients we care for require us to act differently towards them.

Reflective activity

Think about yourself and the things that are important to you. If you were about to be admitted to hospital for an operation, what things would concern you?

We are all individuals with different routines, anxieties and family circumstances. Some of the things you identify might be:

- Will my young son be able to visit?
- Will I be able to have a shower and wash my hair each morning?
- Can I ask questions about things I don't understand without feeling stupid?
- Will I have to share a room with a lot of other people?

The important message here is that the things that are important to us may or may not be as important to others, and the only way we can know is to ask and listen.

This is an important part of the assessment process, which is discussed further in Chapter 3. We also identify assessment as an **enabler** in our model.

Experienced nurses are able to match their actions to these different scenarios without even appearing to stop to think, acting instinctively but still 'getting the job done'. Getting the job done is an important aspect of care delivery in busy clinical areas. Patients now leave hospital earlier, and our increasing knowledge and technology means that we are able to carry out more sophisticated surgery – patients are therefore more critically ill. We need to be able to look after all the patients in our care safely and effectively. Unfortunately that doesn't always leave a lot of time to explain to student nurses what we are doing or why we are doing it.

This chapter aims to help you identify what clinical skills nurses use in care delivery, explore the complexity of that care delivery and start to look at how you might 'unpack' the component parts of skill delivery, in other words be able to identify the separate and discrete elements that 'come together' to make up any clinical skill. Having done this you can start to apply this process to help you develop any new skill. As you will have experienced, sometimes carrying out a skill can look easy when an experienced nurse performs it, but in reality it is more difficult than it looks. Knowing what the separate 'parts' of a skill are goes some way towards not only understanding what is involved in skill delivery but also identifying what areas you need to develop. This is the first step in helping you apply this learning to different situations; we call this transferability of skills.

Keywords

Enabler

Enablers are the essential and underpinning skills that come together to provide expert professional practice.

According to Dunn and Hansford (1997) the part of the programme that helps student nurses learn about clinical practice is one of the 'critical parts of nurse education'. They therefore put the importance on the clinical learning environment, suggesting that it is important not only for learning psychomotor skills but also for 'the development of attitudes, knowledge and clinical problem solving abilities'.

However this 'practice' is difficult to learn. Clinical areas are busy and, although you will work with your **mentor** and other qualified nurses, there are times when you will work with unqualified staff or on your own. So how do you know you are carrying out the care correctly? Not only are clinical areas today busy and patients are more dependent on us for their care, i.e. are unable to look after themselves, but often clinical areas are short-staffed. This makes learning clinical skills difficult at times.

In order to overcome this, most preregistration nursing programmes today try to prepare student nurses for practice by teaching them some clinical skills at university. This usually takes place in a skills laboratory, which is specifically designed for this purpose. While this enables students to have some 'mastery' of skills and practise them in a safe environment before they meet an actual patient, it can mean that students see these skills as separate from each other, rather than as part of 'joined up' care delivery. Also, of course, there is no patient involved and students can find it difficult to act as if there is.

As a result of this, Kleehammer *et al.* (1990) suggest that many students may experience 'reality shock' when they move out of the skills laboratories into clinical areas. Kramer, who is credited with identifying and explaining reality shock, describes it as 'the specific shock-like reactions of new workers when they find themselves in a work situation for which they have spent several years preparing and for which they were going to be prepared and then suddenly find they are not' (Kramer 1974, p. viii).

There are many reasons for this. Opportunities for learning skills may be limited. The student has to adjust to many different clinical environments, including specialist areas. There may be quite some time between being shown a skill and practising it in the clinical arena. Also, in the clinical area students are watched when delivering care, by patients, relatives, nurses and other health care professionals.

It has also been suggested that, unless student nurses have been taught how to transfer this knowledge to actual patient care, they often feel insecure about their skills when they come into contact with patients. Patients may have conditions and/or problems that

Keywords

Mentor

The qualified nurse who is responsible for both facilitating the learning opportunities available for a student nurses and assessing a student nurse during a clinical placement.

mean that clinical skills have to be adapted to meet these needs. Other authors go as far as to suggest that students have to relearn skills because the anxiety they experience when faced with the 'reality' of care may mean that they forget what they have been taught (Nolan and Nolan 1997).

Added to this, student nurses often compare their own practice with more experienced nurses, and this can reinforce a lack of confidence in their own abilities.

This is reflected in some major reports into nursing undertaken recently, in particular *Fitness for Practice* (UKCC 1999), commissioned by the United Kingdom Central Council (nursing's former professional body), and *Making a Difference*, produced by the Department of Health (1999). Both these reports highlighted the importance of clinical skills, and in particular whether students were sufficiently proficient in these skills at the point of qualification. Universities have now amended their nursing programmes in order to make sure that the clinical skill component as part of care delivery is easily identified. However, even this is difficult: nurses' roles change as they take on extra responsibilities and carry out skills traditionally linked with the doctor's role.

In our preregistration nursing programme, those of us involved in teaching clinical skills have expressed the same concerns. We have also questioned how the students 'use' the taught skills in clinical areas. Are students able to alter the way they carry out the skill if they meet a situation they weren't expecting, for example an immobile or confused patient? Also if they need to carry out the skill in a slightly different way, what knowledge did they apply in order to do this safely?

Evaluations completed by students and clinical staff highlight the same concerns. In particular, students identify that they want to be able to act upon and understand the skills they use in practice. As identified earlier, student nurses at the end of the programme often lack confidence and feel unprepared for the transition to qualified nurse.

This is understandable when clinical areas are so busy, patients have quite different needs and care delivery is so multifaceted. Even so, experienced nurses are quick to detect and respond to situations that are often unpredictable. In doing so they are using other 'skills', such as assessment and decision-making.

It is therefore important that clinical skills are not learned in isolation from learning how to care for a patient. Skills are complex and require practice in a variety of settings. Not only are students anxious to acquire these skills but mentors also assess clinical skill delivery when they make a judgement about a student nurse's performance in practice. No wonder, then, that student nurses are anxious about attaining these skills and so it is easy for them to focus on the 'doing', which gives them some confidence in being able to carry out their role effectively, instead of seeing the skill as part of the care package.

What do we mean by clinical skills?

⊶ Keywords

Psychomotor skills
Also referred to as motor skills, these are the nursing actions that we carry out or perform. The term is used in nursing in relation to carrying out a procedure, or series of coordinated steps, when performing a clinical skill.

Often clinical skills are referred to as **'psychomotor' skills**. This is how they were traditionally viewed in nursing, described as this in student nurses' reports, and still described in this way in much of the nursing literature. However, we and some other writers (Bjork and Kirkevold 1999) see this description as being too narrow, as it seems to suggest that it is the performance of the skill that is most important.

We feel that is therefore essential that we provide a definition of what we mean by 'clinical skills' in this context. The word 'skill' suggests practical ability, dexterity, competence, expertise and mastery, which reflects the 'performance'.

For example there is quite a difference between how someone carries out a skill for the first time and a person who has some experience with that skill. If we apply this to someone making a cake for the first time, there are lots of 'parts' of the skill to learn. There is a recipe to follow, ingredients to weigh out. Other 'underpinning' skills to learn such as 'creaming' the butter and sugar together, exercising judgement as to whether the cake mixture is of the right consistency, how much fluid to add, choosing the appropriate cake tin and judging whether the cake is properly cooked. The 'skilled' cook does not have to use a recipe, can judge weights, consistency and whether the cake is cooked almost instinctively, thus demonstrating the practical ability, dexterity, competence, expertise and mastery identified above.

Farley and Hendry (1997, p. 2) reinforce this and suggest that: 'a skill is action oriented, but it also requires an element of thought. A skill should bring together both theory and practice – it is not just about being able to do something, but about understanding the rationale that underpins the action'.

Bjork and Kirkevold (1999) support this, stating that when clinical skills are referred to as psychomotor skills it suggests a limited understanding of practical skills in nursing. They go on to comment that in nursing we still place value on the 'speed and enactment of certain motor steps', judging them as 'the parameters of skilled action'. Bjork (1999) suggests that clinical skills ought to be thought of as actions relating to 'the patients' physical comfort, hygiene and safe medical treatment' but clearly states that 'good nursing' not only involves the physical and technical aspects of care delivery but also demands that these should be merged with the psychosocial elements.

According to Bjork and Kirkevold (1999) this is skilled behaviour, which is complex and is not only about 'doing' but also becomes more polished throughout the doing, in response to the needs of the patient and the clinical context. They suggest that the delivery of these skills is sophisticated and a deliberate consequence of the nurse interpreting cues, and that nurses underpin this skill delivery not only with their knowledge of the patient but also with theory and ethical knowledge. This further supports the notion that when carrying out clinical skills the patients' needs are fundamental. Nurses need to consider not only how to respond to these needs but also how they relate to the patient. Bjork and Kirkvold (1999) therefore conclude that an essential part of any skill is 'caring', which they suggest involves 'relating to the person as a human being worthy of respect and thoughtfulness'. This principle is also supported by Staib (2003), who states that nursing is about providing care, which is more than a 'series of tasks', and involves demonstrating a 'caring attitude' while performing skills. She states that this is concerned with a 'genuine concern for patients' welfare'.

One of the reasons that clinical skills have traditionally been thought of as just the 'doing' aspect of care is that traditionally nursing was 'explained' as comprising three types (domains) of knowledge: cognitive (the knowledge required), psychomotor (the doing) and affective (attitudes), and so these were separated whereas they should be integrated.

> ## ✍ *Over to you*
>
> Consider what has been said about the domains of nursing knowledge above. Can you think of a clinical skill you have practised and identify not only how you did it (psychomotor), but also the underpinning knowledge and the interpersonal skills required to carry it out?

So what do we mean by skills? How can we 'break down' care into its essential 'nuts and bolts' (components) to explore the complexity and diversity of care delivery? Why focus on psychomotor skills – this puts the emphasis on 'doing' without knowing?

The term 'clinical skill' seems to be interpreted as something that we carry out instead of the process of care delivery. We want to challenge that notion and help you to think about skills from a broader perspective.

There are two processes involved in this, first understanding what these skills are and secondly 'unpacking' the individual 'enabling' skills in care delivery in order to put them back together to make a meaningful whole in different situations.

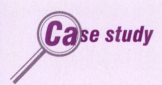

Mary Wood – caring for the whole patient

Mary Wood is a fit lady of 82 years. Having retired from her job as a headmistress, she has been an active member of the local community. She is an avid golfer, playing every Friday. She bakes and runs a cake stall for the WRVS once a month. She also happily uses her time to undertake duties of shopping and driving for those who are less independent than herself.

She underwent waiting list surgery yesterday for removal of a benign lump (lipoma) from her lower back. This morning she is very quiet and lethargic, so Tracy, her primary nurse, suggests that she helps Mary to get washed and changed into a clean nightie to make her more comfortable.

While washing Mary, Tracy asks some general questions about how Mary is feeling. She asks them quietly and manages to convey some genuine concern for Mary's answers. She notices that Mary finds some movements difficult. She also notes the vagueness of some of Mary's answers and the fact that Mary looks pale and anxious. She decides to ask Mary if she is worried about anything,

Mary then starts to cry. She confesses that she has had a sleepless night. She has had some pain and difficulty with some movement since her operation, which hasn't responded to painkillers, and she is scared that won't be able to cope at home without help, thus becoming dependent on others like her friends.

Tracy is able to reassure Mary that what she is feeling is usual for her condition and that her pain and impaired movement will improve. She also says she will get in touch with the doctor straight away to review her prescription.

Carrying out a bed bath is one of the most intimate tasks that the nurse performs. It not only allows us to help maintain the patient's hygiene needs but also provides an opportunity to observe for physical (rashes, bruising), psychological (anxiety) and social (embarrassment) well being.

Tracy employed some sophisticated skills of assessment, observation, interpretation, decision-making, communication and interpersonal skills in this example.

What conclusions would you have drawn from Mary's reactions?

The case study above should have helped you to see what individual (or discrete) skills underpin any aspect of care or skill delivery. We felt it would be useful to start to identify what we believe are the essential components of care delivery. We came to the conclusion that to focus on clinical skills in a traditional way, such as blood pressure measurement, for example, would be limiting and not effectively reflect the complex nature of the delivery of nursing care today. Nurses need to have the skills to respond appropriately to what Edwards (2003) describes as an 'unpredictable environment'.

We felt that even calling these activities clinical skills was restrictive; that it would lead us to think about skills in a narrow way. We decided that using the term 'skills for practice' was an easier way of understanding what we do, and that these skills for practice would include:

- Assessment
- Comfort/caring
- Clinical skills
- Communicating and interacting with patients
- Health and safety
- Organisational skills
- Personal and professional development.

We now need to give you our rationale for classifying skills in this way.

Assessment

Assessment is not only part of skill delivery but is also a complex skill. It is a skill that is difficult for students to master, as it requires a sound knowledge base. However, knowledge in itself is limited if we don't have the appropriate communication and interpersonal skills to obtain information from patients and relatives to enable us to make sure that our nursing interventions are suitable to meet the patient's individual needs. This individualised approach is dependent on us being able to also use skills of observation, measurement, interpretation, prioritising and decision-making. The skill of assessment is therefore discussed further in Chapter 3.

Comfort and caring

Comfort and caring are very broad categories, and therefore not easy to explain, but important nevertheless. Most of us would identify these as being a key part of nursing, and patients would also identify these as essential.

Many writers have discussed their significance and attempted to explain them. Gorham (1962), for example, recognises that, although patients place importance on nurses helping them meet their basic care needs such as hygiene, they also felt it was important for nurses to be able to promote comfort. Bjork and Kirkvold (1999) and Staib (2003) both agree that caring is fundamental to care delivery.

We felt that good examples in this category would be 'caring for the patient in pain', 'promoting continence', 'promoting sleep' and 'caring for the dying patient'. These are essential elements of nursing care, but complex and themselves made up of lots of individual skills, such as, for example communication, assessment and administration of medicines, to name but a few.

Because these are difficult concepts to understand we take an example in Chapter 4, and discuss it in detail, to help explain more fully our approach to 'skills for practice' development. We have chosen to look at 'helping a patient meet their nutritional needs'. This is an example of an area of nursing care that is currently attracting a lot of attention, in the media, nursing and Department of Health reports. The reason for this is that it has been an area that is misunderstood and has been done badly (Burke 1997). Exploring this skill and all its discrete elements will help us identify where the gaps in our knowledge and skills base are.

Clinical skills

Although we have suggested that this is a rather narrow way of looking at skills, we felt there were some nursing activities that we could call clinical skills. Certainly if you talk about clinical skills to other nursing colleagues they can easily identify some nursing activities, such as giving injections and changing wound dressings, that are a fundamental part of patient care. Other examples of clinical skills could include those that we refer to as 'observations' such as blood pressure measurement and recording temperature, pulse and respiratory rates.

Communicating and interacting with patients

While communication is fundamental to any skill delivery, there are examples of specific communications with patients/families that could be said to 'stand alone' – for example, providing patients with information about their medication, forthcoming operation or X-ray investigation. Other examples might be providing health information, such as advice on stopping smoking or managing diets, or responding to 'difficult' patients or situations, e.g. the patient who is confused, in pain, anxious or aggressive, or has been robbed of speech by a stroke.

Health and safety

We use this category to include those skills that are required to be updated yearly, such as moving and handling, cardiopulmonary resuscitation, disposal of hazardous substances and sharps, and food handling. We also felt that we should identify other skills that we recommend should be revisited at least yearly to maintain safe practice, for example administration of medicines and infection control procedures. These skills are usually incorporated into Trust policies. These policy documents will indicate requirements for updating, including training.

Organisational skills

Student nurses sometimes fail to recognise the skills that nurses must possess in order to manage patient care effectively, whether that be the management of an individual patient's care, the care of a group of patients or management of a clinical area. In our experience these are skills that students find difficult, particularly as they move out of one role, being used to being directed, to that of the one directing others' actions as a more senior student or qualified nurse. Some examples in this category would be conducting handovers, delegation, prioritisation and time management. An important part of organising care is coordinating the input of other health care professionals, which involves the nurse communicating with, and working as part of, a multidisciplinary team. Working with the multidisciplinary team involves other skills – the 'softer' skills that relate to the self. Examples of these would be assertiveness, communication and negotiation skills, which are discussed later, in Chapter 5.

Personal and professional development

We thought in this category we wouldn't identify the skills but would encourage individual students to identify to the skills they wish to develop. Perhaps there is a 'gap' in the student's personal development, such as the 'soft' skills identified above, or a skill they wish to master in a variety of settings. These could be related to the clinical context in which they plan to work as qualified nurses. Examples of these skills could be undertaking venepuncture and cannulation. These are skills previously associated with qualified nurses in a specialist role but more recently are expected of all qualified nurses and are being introduced into preregistration nursing programmes.

Venepuncture and cannulation, as well as some of the skills identified in the other categories, are explored in Chapter 4.

⊶ᴨ *Keywords*

Evidence-based practice
A way of working that relies on you retrieving and using information from a variety of sources to underpin your practice, particularly research, audit, clinical guidelines and service user opinion. This needs to be constantly updated to provide contemporary 'best' practice.

Contemporary nursing care

Before undertaking any skill it is important to identify the underpinning knowledge required to perform that skill safely and with understanding. Contemporary nursing care is **evidence-based practice**; this means that nurses must know the rationale for the delivery of care in a certain way, based upon research and experience. The care we deliver should always be up to date and clearly underpinned by theory. This may involve appropriate positioning, knowledge of anatomy, use of specialist equipment, knowledge of trust policies, consideration of ethical and legal implications, etc. So being well informed before starting is crucial.

Kramer (1978) states that, because real situations are complex, 'students need to experience the causes and effects of their actions and solve problems'. This supports what our students have identified, that they need to 'understand why' as well as 'knowing how' in order to be able to adapt their skills in response to patient needs and different clinical environments. This requires a sound knowledge base.

Underpinning skills

The care we deliver and the skills we perform always have a patient as the focus. It is important to think about the best way of delivering care for that individual based upon their care/therapeutic needs. You also need to consider the beliefs and information needs of the patient and the context in which the skill is to be carried out. We always need to be aware of health and safety issues, both for the patients in our care and for ourselves. In other words, the nurse should work within Trust policies, professional guidelines such as the Nursing and Midwifery Council's (2002) Code of Professional Conduct, and government legislation.

When dealing with patients we must be aware of their anxieties and needs, particularly for information and support. Carrying out a skill involves obtaining the patient's consent, information-giving, reassurance and maintaining patient comfort, privacy and dignity. Therefore good interpersonal skills, communication skills and a **professional** attitude are very important in the delivery of care.

Learning clinical skills

So far we have tried to encourage you to see skills for practice as requiring good theoretical underpinning, constant updating and to be adapted to individual patient needs. What makes care delivery so diverse is that 'nurses encounter situations daily that do not fit with previous experience' (Staib 2003) and therefore you will need to constantly review your own practice. Clinical skills are not easily acquired: the types of skill required by today's nurses are changing and becoming more complicated, and there is an expectation that student nurses have some understanding of the care they deliver. The types of skill we perform change as nursing roles evolve, and

Keywords

Professional

Nurses are expected in act in a professional way when dealing with patients. This involves maintaining patient confidentiality, demonstrating a non-judgemental attitude and maintaining the patient's privacy and dignity. It also assumes that nurses will accept responsibility and accountability for their actions. In some situations it will involve acting for the patient as their advocate, when patients are unable to make an informed decision for themselves.

you need to think about how you will learn the new skills that you may need in the future.

One of the most significant and recent developments in preregistration nursing was Project 2000 (UKCC 1986). This was an attempt to overcome some well-documented 'shortfalls' in nurse education, which included skill development. One of the key outcomes of Project 2000 was the need for the nurse to be a 'knowledgeable doer' and also to carry out skills confidently.

Loveridge (2003, p. 36) uses the work of Sloboda (1993) to explain that confidence in skill delivery involves 'fluency (an integrated sequence), rapidity (the speed that tasks are carried out), automaticity (the ease of approach), simultaneity (the ability to perform other tasks at the same time), and the knowledge that is readily available and relevant. All require practice.'

To make this clearer we could consider what is involved when we move a patient from bed to chair. Obviously, to maintain the safety of patients, colleagues and ourselves we need to carry out the manoeuvre as efficiently as possible.

- **Fluency** would involve making the move as 'smooth' and controlled as possible to ensure patient safety and comfort. We need to be able to carry out the stages of the move in the right order, but also to be able to see the whole skill rather than just a series of steps.

- **Rapidity**: Carrying out the move too slowly might compromise nurse safety while moving too quickly might compromise patient safety and cause distress to the patient.

- **Automaticity** suggests that the nurse is knowledgeable about, and is competent to perform the move, which would involve considering (assessing) the needs of the patient and being knowledgeable about the type of equipment to be used.

- **Simultaneity**: Being able to note several things concurrently; observing the patient to note discomfort, ease of movement or anxiety. Also being aware of colleague's movements and assessing the environment for obstacles.

- **Knowledge** would include topics such as ergonomics, anatomy and physiology of bones and joints, health and safety principles, Trust policy, resources and current approved moves and equipment.

Learning skills for practice therefore involves not just the repetition of a skill, but identifying and using patient information, considering the context, i.e. specific area of practice, reflecting on our experience and considering our strengths and weaknesses.

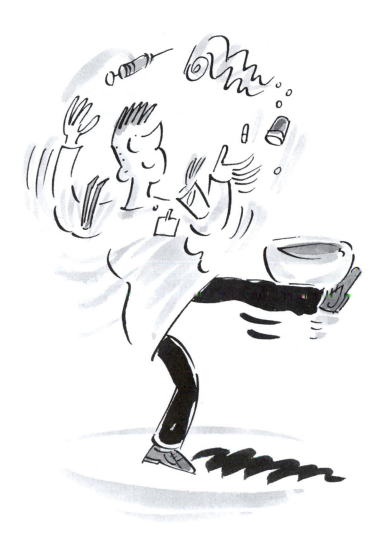

I thought I was learning to be a nurse, not a juggler!

Competent
Possessing the necessary knowledge and skill to carry out nursing care.

Reflection
'Thinking back' about an activity or situation in order to make sense of it and consider how we might alter how we do things in the future – in other words, a way of learning from experience.

This example demonstrates that in order to become **competent** we need to 'unpack' the individual skills in care delivery in order to put them back together to make a meaningful whole in different situations. To be successful we need to encourage **reflection**, problem solving and decision-making.

This is summed up by Edwards (2003), who states that in order 'to deal effectively with rapid change we need to become skilled in higher-level thinking', for example analysis and interpretation. Chapter 2 will explore this. It will identify what the basic components of skill development are, discuss what makes learning effective and introduce you to a template for skill development.

One important aspect of learning is the knowledge, previous experience, beliefs and values that we bring with us. This might be personal experience of being ill, or looking after children or relatives. It could be life or job experience, dealing with difficult customers in a bar, or being responsible for a group of staff in a shop. These experiences will 'shape' our view of nursing and caring and will provide us with some skills to apply in new and different contexts. This personal and professional knowledge therefore underpins and 'shapes' the kind of practitioner you become.

How this affects you

Often, using diagrams can help us think of the way in which several concepts fit together. Throughout this book we will ask you to think of clinical skills as more than 'doing' tasks or procedures.

Think about the way that tissue fluid and blood maintain the correct balance of oxygen and nutrients received by cells, and their role in removing waste products from the cells, so helping them to function. Can you remember or imagine what it's like to stand in a ward and not understand what the staff are doing? You can't understand the jargon they use. You might feel that you can't function as a member of the ward team until someone starts to explain things. They need to show you how to do things and/or get you to read about the care they deliver in that environment. As such you will require different types of knowledge to develop your skills, so that you can function in clinical environments that are supportive for patients and optimise health.

Any living environment is complex and constantly adapting to change and therefore can seem a little chaotic at times. When we are new to the environment we like structure and guidance – remember how useful a map can be in a city you've never visited before. Physiologically there are lots of feedback loops to ensure that our bodies are kept as stable and healthy as possible. A framework can provide the same kind of stability: identify what you know, how you performed and what else you'd need to know for the next time or the next patient. It is a way to cope with complexity.

Finally the source of the oxygen, nutrition and defence mechanism for a cell relies on the circulatory system. It's a fundamental system without which the cell wouldn't be viable. Think about a tissue that's deprived of oxygen (e.g. pressure-damaged skin) – the circulation is compromised, stops functioning appropriately and then the skin dies. You could start to see your knowledge base in this light. You are provided with different types of knowledge and information, either at university, college or in clinical placement and work environments. This needs to be processed,

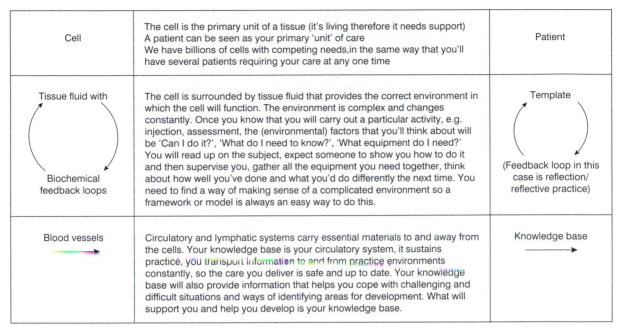

Cell	The cell is the primary unit of a tissue (it's living therefore it needs support) A patient can be seen as your primary 'unit' of care We have billions of cells with competing needs, in the same way that you'll have several patients requiring your care at any one time	Patient
Tissue fluid with Biochemical feedback loops	The cell is surrounded by tissue fluid that provides the correct environment in which the cell will function. The environment is complex and changes constantly. Once you know that you will carry out a particular activity, e.g. injection, assessment, the (environmental) factors that you'll think about will be 'Can I do it?', 'What do I need to know?', 'What equipment do I need?' You will read up on the subject, expect someone to show you how to do it and then supervise you, gather all the equipment you need together, think about how well you've done and what you'd do differently the next time. You need to find a way of making sense of a complicated environment so a framework or model is always an easy way to do this.	Template (Feedback loop in this case is reflection/ reflective practice)
Blood vessels	Circulatory and lymphatic systems carry essential materials to and away from the cells. Your knowledge base is your circulatory system, it sustains practice, you transport information to and from practice environments constantly, so the care you deliver is safe and up to date. Your knowledge base will also provide information that helps you cope with challenging and difficult situations and ways of identifying areas for development. What will support you and help you develop is your knowledge base.	Knowledge base

Figure 1.1 *Circulation and skills.*

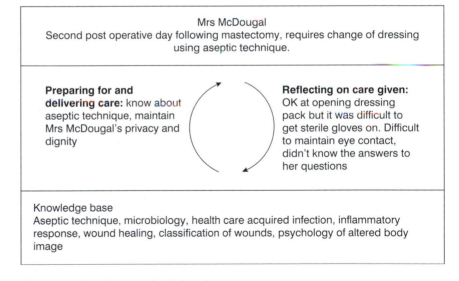

Figure 1.2 *Applying the circulation diagram.*

stored and then transported and used by you when you deliver care. If you do not develop and update your knowledge base, your clinical care will not be viable. It will be damaged, compromised and you'll stop functioning appropriately, i.e. your evidence base for practice will be weak/non-existent. That will not be good for patients or for yourself as a professional.

Conclusions

Care delivery is complex and involves a range of skills. Learning skills for practice is a vital element of care delivery, and the skills themselves are dynamic, involving refinement and responsiveness by the nurse to ever-changing patient circumstances and clinical environments.

RRRRRR*Rapid recap*

Check your progress so far by working through each of the following questions.

1. What 'key' skills do you need to draw on to deliver individualised and holistic care?
2. What knowledge and understanding do you need to 'perform' a skill to an acceptable standard that ensures patient safety, comfort and dignity?
3. What 'categories' of skills do nurses require to deliver care?

If you have difficulty with more than one of the questions, read through the section again to refresh your understanding before moving on.

References

Bjork, I.T. (1999) Practical skill development in new nurses. *Nursing Inquiry*, **6**, 34–47.

Bjork, I.T. and Kirkevold, M. (1999) Issues in nurses' practical skill development in the clinical setting. *Journal of Nursing Care Quality*, **14**, 72–84.

Burke, A. (1997) *Hungry in Hospital?* Association of Community Health Councils of England and Wales, London.

Department of Health (1999) *Making a Difference. Strengthening the nursing, midwifery and health visiting contribution to health and healthcare*. The Stationery Office, London.

Dunn, S.V. and Hansford, B. (1997) Undergraduate nursing students' perceptions of their clinical learning environment. *Journal of Advanced Nursing*, **25**, 1299–1306.

Edwards, S. (2003) Critical thinking at the bedside: a practical perspective. *British Journal of Nursing*, **12**, 1142–1149.

Farley, A. and Hendry, C. (1997) Teaching practical skills: a guide for preceptors. *Nursing Standard*, **11**(29), 46–48.

Gorham, W.A. (1962) Staff nursing behaviours contributing to patient care and improvement. *Nursing Research*, **11**, 68–70.

Kleehammer, K., Hart, A.L. and Keck, J.F. (1990) Nursing students' perceptions of anxiety-producing situations in the clinical setting. *Journal of Nursing Education*, **29**, 183–187.

Kramer, M. (1974) *Reality Shock. Why nurses leave nursing*. C.V. Mosby, St Louis, MO.

Kramer, M. (1978) Role conception of baccalaureate nurses and success in hospital nursing. *Nursing Research*, **15**, 428–439.

Loveridge, N. (2003) Acquiring percussion and auscultation skills. *Emergency Nurse*, **11**, 31–39.

Nolan, J. and Nolan, M. (1997) Self directed and student-centred learning in nursing education. *British Journal of Nursing*, **6**, 51–55.

Nursing and Midwifery Council (2002) *Code of Professional Conduct: Standards for conduct, performance and ethics*. Nursing and Midwifery Council, London.

Sloboda, J. (1993) What is skill and how is it acquired? In: Loveridge, N. (2003) Acquiring percussion and auscultation skills. *Emergency Nurse*, **11**, 31.

Staib, S. (2003) Teaching and measuring critical thinking. *Journal of Nursing Education*, **42**, 498.

UKCC (1986) *Project 2000: A new preparation for practice*. United Kingdom Central Council for Nursing, Midwifery and Health Visiting, London.

UKCC (1999) *Fitness for Practice. The UKCC Commission for Nursing and Midwifery Education*. United Kingdom Central Council for Nursing, Midwifery and Health Visiting, London.

2

Learning clinical skills

Learning outcomes

By the end of this chapter you should be able to:

- Explain the term 'reflection'
- Link the contribution of 'thinking skills' to the development of patient care
- Identify the rationale for recognising individual learning styles
- Describe how we can learn from practice.

🔑 Keywords

Template
A guide for how to carry out something.

Introducing a new approach to learning about skills

In the last chapter we talked about the need to 'unpack' a skill in order to learn it. This chapter has been written to try and provide you with a 'toolbox', which we refer to as a **template**, to learn any new skill you come across and enable you to transfer knowledge and abilities to a new situation. We talk more about this template in Chapter 4; here we want to focus on the way in which we learn and relate it to skill development and mastery. The first step you need to take is to think about yourself and how you learn, and compare this with what other authors say about learning.

When we introduced our 'circulation diagram' in Chapter 1 (Figure 1.2, p. 15), we used the example of changing a wound dressing to suggest where the gaps in your knowledge might be – for example a difficulty in putting gloves on or answering questions, both of which you would need to find out more about. The diagram also highlighted the fact that you will already have some knowledge, the knowledge you bring with you to any new situation.

When carrying out an aseptic technique such as changing a wound dressing, you might start by thinking about the 'steps' you should take in order to do it correctly, such as:

- Wash hands
- Prepare equipment
- Provide an explanation to the patient

and so on.

Breaking down a skill into its parts (or components) is not a new idea. In fact, that's the way you probably already go about learning a skill (as identified above), although you might not be aware of it. This is commented upon by many writers, for example Patricia Benner (1984) who has identified the 'journey' that takes a nurse from novice (student) to expert (qualified nurse). She uses a model developed by Dreyfus and Dreyfus (1980), which describes five levels of skill 'proficiency': novice, advanced beginner, competent, proficient and expert. Benner (1984) describes how the student initially learns about skills as a series of steps or 'rules', which makes them 'limited' and 'inflexible'. It isn't until the student acquires some experience of the clinical area that they are able to see the 'whole' picture and start to use this experience to make judgements about the care they are delivering – proficiency.

When we break learning a skill down into steps using our template we identify the parts as being:

- A definition/explanation of what it is you are trying to do – **What is it?**
- A rationale for what you are doing – **Why do it?**
- What you need to know in order to do it – **Knowledge underpinning practice**
- **How to do it**
- Sources of information – **Reference list**

and

- **Reflection** on how you did.

> ### Over to you
>
> Take some time here to think about a skill you have recently acquired, taking and recording a pulse, for example. Using the template above try to identify some responses related to taking and recording a pulse rate.

The complexity of skill delivery in practice

Now, think about the reality of the clinical situation and patients you have nursed. Consider the patient who has plaster casts on both arms. How would you record their pulse? What about the patient who is too confused to cooperate? How would you manage this situation?

If you record a faster or slower than expected pulse rate, what would your conclusions be? For example, could the patient have undertaken recent exercise, taken medication that alters heart rate, or recently returned from theatre? Has the patient got an infection, in which case what else would the patient be complaining of?

We have suggested some explanations for an altered pulse rate, but how would you find out the answers to questions like these? They are based on knowledge and experience, but first you need to know what the normal range for the pulse rate is, the location of pulse sites, how we describe a pulse, and explanations for a fast/slow/irregular/thready pulse. You also need to know what questions to ask, in order to identify the gaps in your knowledge. We have shown you how using our template would have helped you ask questions to identify the information you need.

The next step is more difficult; this is identifying the significance of your findings. You need to decide why the patient is exhibiting a fast pulse rate so that you know what questions to ask, or what other observations to take.

Underpinning skills

The example outlined above is a typical one. Patients very often have several health problems, making a complex situation. Patients don't only have physical needs to be met, they also require explanations (information needs) and reassurance (psychological needs). They should have their privacy and dignity (social needs) respected and be made comfortable after an observation or procedure. This is the 'whole' picture, based on much more than just the 'doing' of the skill. The delivery of holistic care acknowledges the psychological, social, spiritual and physical needs of the patient.

Holistic care delivery, because it views the patient as an individual with their own unique needs, requires what Antrobus (1997) refers to as 'sophisticated' skills such as critical thinking. Therefore, essential to good skill development and holistic care are problem-solving, and the exercise of professional judgement built upon reflection, critical thinking and decision-making

In other words you need to use 'thinking' skills to acknowledge that the patient in front of you is reacting differently or has other health care needs. Which means they may not reflect the 'textbook' example you have been taught and shown. This then involves you in a decision based upon an assessment of the situation of how you might 'adapt' the skill or procedure for this patient.

One important aspect of skill development then is reflection. What did you do that was different from the expected procedure? How did you make your decision? What sources of knowledge did you use to 'inform' your decision? What do you need to do now to ensure that you feel confident when performing the skill next time, perhaps in a different situation again?

Reflection

We have already identified that clinical situations are complex, patients' conditions change quickly and they may have more than one disease process, which is compounded often by complicated treatments. Also patients don't always behave the way you expect them to. This kind of situation can appear very muddled and confusing to new student nurses. Decisions made by qualified nurses may be difficult to understand, and looking for answers in books and journals doesn't always help as they can't take into account the aspects of the patient that are personal to them. Reflection is a means of exploring an experience we have had in order to understand it. When we undertake reflection deliberately to help our understanding, by 'thinking back' about a situation we have been involved in, this is usually referred to as 'reflection on action' (Schon 1983). This type of reflection is usually where we start as new learners, and involves us in actively examining our experiences by asking ourselves questions and drawing conclusions. It can be useful to undertake this type of reflection with others, to develop 'shared understandings' of situations.

When we have referred to the way experienced nurses function, we have identified that they are able to respond to changes in the patient's situation and amend the care they deliver accordingly. This 'conscious' reflection involving interpreting and making decisions as we go along is referred to as 'reflection in action', and requires both experience and a good knowledge base. Schon (1983) explains this as 'thinking on your feet'.

By 'reflecting' on your performance in this way you can start to develop a range of other skills identified previously – problem-solving, critical thinking and decision-making – to enhance your learning. In other words, you can start to develop the ability to use and apply the knowledge across a range of clinical situations.

However, reflection is not an easy process to master, and one reason why students like yourselves may find it difficult is that writers define it in different ways. Dewey (1933), one of the first to describe reflection, identifies it as 'the turning over of a subject in the mind and giving it serious and consecutive consideration'. He suggested that it involved emotions as well as critical thinking and emotions. Reflection involves us in moving away from acceptance of information (which we do as 'novices') to questioning and becoming active in our own learning (Glaze 2002). Many other writers (Schon 1983, Boud *et al.* 1985, Mezirow 1990) take this further, clearly identifying reflection as a learning tool.

Brookfield (1995) believes that the value of reflection is that we can underpin our actions with a rationale. This rationale is based upon making connections between theory and practice. By exploring situations and producing explanations we can acknowledge not only that theory should underpin practice but also that theory can emerge from practice. It helps us deal with challenges. Reflection is not an easy process and is one that new student nurses find difficult, so many writers, for example Gibbs (1988), have developed strategies or frameworks for using reflection, which usually centre on a series of questions or tasks.

If you wish to know more about reflection, there is another book in this series written by Melanie Jasper, *Beginning Reflective Practice* (2003), which you might find useful.

The importance of using reflection in skill development is that it can move you as the learner from technical expertise (skill proficiency) to interpreting, i.e. making sense of the clinical situation or context, and help you to develop critical thinking skills (Chandler 2000). Critical thinking is a process that involves investigation, links reflection with 'informed action' but also has an affective (emotive) ingredient. Brookfield (2000) suggests that linking feelings and knowledge is crucial to the process of critical thinking. Critical thinking is discussed in more detail later in this chapter.

In order to be able to make judgements, we need to undertake a reflective process. However, if this process is to be critical it requires us to have 'affective learning and ways of knowing'. Ruth-Sahd (2003) suggests this critical reflection should involve affective ways of knowing to help us deal with 'uncertainty and conflict'. She suggests that exploring feelings and emotions can powerfully shape reflection. Later in the chapter we look at different approaches to learning and introduce the notion of intuition as a way of explaining how we 'know' something.

Problem solving

An approach used more and more in preregistration programmes is that of problem-based learning. In our university we use the term 'enquiry-based learning', as students get involved in their own learning by identifying what they don't know and then finding out the information. The first step therefore is to identify and explore the problem. This is a very useful strategy for students of nursing to engage in as it is very closely linked to the nursing process and its stages of assessment, planning, implementation and evaluation, used regularly in clinical areas.

For example, using the nursing process the nurse would collect information about the patient by asking questions of them or their relatives, recording observations, reading case note, etc. (assessment). They would then identify the nursing care the patient requires, taking into account nursing interventions, staff and equipment needed (planning). The next stages are carrying out the care (implementation) and then reviewing how successful the nursing interventions were (evaluation).

The starting point is identifying the problem.

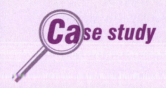

Case study

Dot Sugden – identifying the problem

Dot Sugden is 74 years old and usually enjoys good health, although she is underweight for her age and height. She lives alone in a small one-bedroom bungalow, having moved there 2 years ago after the death of her husband. Her son visited her yesterday and was shocked to find his mother very confused, in her nightdress in the middle of the afternoon and looking unwell. The GP visited and noted that Dot was displaying signs of dehydration. It was very difficult to obtain any information from Dot and so, given her general condition, the GP arranged admission to a medical ward for investigation.

You assist your mentor to assess Dot on admission. Her observations are checked, revealing a weak pulse of 58 bpm, and a blood pressure measurement of 100/60 mmHg. She has a temperature of 39.2°C.

The only medication Dot takes is digoxin 62.5 mcg daily, having been diagnosed as having 'atrial fibrillation' almost 10 years earlier. Otherwise there is nothing of note in her past medical history.

You note that your mentor palpates Dot's abdomen. The assessment form contains information about Dot's sunken eyes and dry skin.

Your mentor asks if you will try to encourage Dot to drink, to record all input and output carefully and to try to obtain a midstream specimen of urine (MSU).

This is a very common scenario in nursing, as patients rarely present with only one problem or disease process. It is also complicated, although for the experienced nurse there are lots of clues.

Where would you start in trying to understand this situation? Firstly you need to identify all the areas you are unclear about in order to research them. The next step is to try and put the separate pieces of information together.

Over to you

Ask yourself the following questions:
- What parts of the scenario don't you understand?
- Where can you find the information you need to answer your questions?

- What do you understand by the term 'dehydration'?
- Do Dot's observations fall within the norms for her age group?
- What is the relevance of the comments about Dot's eyes and skin?
- Why would your mentor palpate Dot's abdomen – what would this indicate?
- Why would your mentor ask you to encourage drinks and request an MSU?
- What would we be expecting to see reflected on the fluid balance chart?
- What could have caused Dot's confusion?

These questions should be enough to get you started in identifying what the potential problems are. Obviously this kind of questioning requires some skill and experience, but if you undertake this kind of exercise often enough it becomes 'second nature' so that you go through the process without even thinking about it.

Critical thinking

The case study above highlights the fact that carrying out care in clinical situations often involves us in making decisions, and making them quickly, usually without a full set of facts or information. Critical thinking helps us to be more effective in these situations, by involving us in exploring the situation and distinguishing between knowledge and feelings (Price 2004).

Critical thinking is therefore essential to decision-making and is an important skill for qualified nurses to possess as it is now considered to be a routine part of their role (Miller 1992). However, critical thinking is in itself a complex activity, which can be defined as: 'an attitude and a reasoning process involving a number of intellectual skills – a purposeful activity in which ideas are produced and evaluated and judgements made' (Wilkinson 1992).

It involves identifying the beliefs, knowledge and experiences that underpin your actions (what you can assume having met the situation before, or what you know about it). However, Brookfield (1995) suggests that nurses aren't always critical because they base decisions on assumptions without even realising it, and that these assumptions can be flawed. For example the nurse may assume how a patient feels, or assume that the patient does not have severe pain because they appear to be resting. You therefore need to be aware of this and analyse these 'assumptions', taking into account the circumstances in which the situation has arisen, acknowledging the gaps in your knowledge and experience and reviewing and deciding the implications of potential actions (Brookfield 1987).

If we use the case study, we can identify that the mentor's knowledge in this situation could be related to how the ageing process results in reduced circulatory fluid. Her experience would tell her that the elderly are often reluctant to drink, perhaps because it results in more frequent trips to the toilet. This lady has a high temperature, which the mentor would know could cause confusion. She may believe that the confusion might also lead to a further reduction in Dot's fluid intake, and assume, because she analyses these factors, that the most likely cause of Dot's high temperature is a urinary infection.

To explore this idea further, the process of critical thinking involves asking questions such as 'Why do we do it this way?' We have to look at the context (or place) where practice takes place to see how this influences the beliefs and opinions of the staff in that area, and consider the alternatives available to us – what are the other ways of doing this? Possibly we may even reject the usual course of action and ask whether it is still appropriate or 'valid' – is there an evidence base to confirm that this is the best way of dealing with this problem, or is there some new research or evidence relating to this area? Are we carrying out a procedure because it has always been done this way, even when our common sense or experience tells us that there must be a better way of doing it? In other words, critical thinking 'is the art of thinking about your thinking while you are thinking in order to make your thinking better' (Paul 1992).

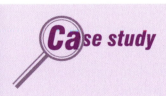

Case study

Keywords

Iatrogenic

Some forms of ill health are caused by treatment – consider the toxic effects of anticancer drugs for example. This is called iatrogenic illness, which comes from the Greek iatro, meaning 'doctor', and genesis, meaning 'origin'.

Laura Jones – the importance of point of view

Laura Jones, aged 36 years, has been admitted this morning to review the treatment for her rheumatoid arthritis. She has had the condition since her late twenties. Laura places a lot of importance on her physical appearance, usually being perfectly made up and wearing expensive nightwear. This is despite continual pain and stiffness in her hands.

Today, however, she is wearing no make up and looks pale and drawn. Although she is responding well to her disease-modifying anti-rheumatoid drugs (DMARDs), her pain is not well controlled and she is experiencing overwhelming tiredness. She is prescribed diclofenac (a non-steroidal anti-inflammatory drug) for her pain relief.

During the afternoon, you get the opportunity to sit and talk to Laura. She tells you that she is unhappy with having to take so many drugs, that she feels they are 'poisoning her system' and 'they don't work anyway, so what is the point?'

You have some sympathy for her point of view, having recently read about **iatrogenic** disease, and wonder whether there are any alternative approaches to her pain relief.

Tony, the physiotherapist who links with the ward, visits later and you ask him if he can suggest some alternative pain relief. He suggests that you both meet with the rheumatoid nurse specialist to 'share' experience and ideas so that you can offer some alternatives to Laura.

What you should be able to see from the case study is that the way we feel about treatments for pain, or our beliefs about the experience of pain, will influence our approach to care. For example, you might be committed to complementary approaches to care, hence your sympathy for Laura's view about drugs poisoning her system. Alternatively you might have difficulty in believing that she is in continual pain, given her appearance.

This is only one perspective. Talking to nurse specialists who have a wealth of knowledge that is clearly based upon experience and evidence can help us understand other types of approach, including the importance of involving patients in the decision-making, moving away from 'Doctor knows best'.

New nurses and experienced qualified nurses approach clinical reasoning (engaging in the discussion process) and critical thinking differently. This is because understanding your experiences is the first step to developing 'thinking' skills. Critical thinking should therefore not only involve cognitive (thinking) skills linked to affective (feelings) skills but should clearly relate to, or emerge from, practice (Benner *et al.* 1996).

If you consider the process outlined above you will see it is very closely linked to reflection; therefore learning to think critically will help us learn to reflect.

Decision-making

Decisions can only be made effectively if we have considered all the alternatives, having investigated what options are available to us and the appropriateness of those options, given the situation we find ourselves in, using the skills identified previously.

Having been involved in making a decision it is important that as student nurses you reflect on the decision, identifying what you did right and learning from your experience. You need to ask questions about the experience, for example those identified in our template, in order to understand what is happening, by asking questions such as 'What do I need know?' and 'How can I find the answers?' These are the questions you would be encouraged to ask if you were undertaking enquiry-based learning, knowing *why* rather than knowing *what*. This in time will help you become more confident.

Learning styles

Mezirow (1991), when explaining how adults (as opposed to children) learn, suggests that they bring to the learning experience, among other things, their underpinning beliefs, learning style and ways of feeling. He goes on to state that learners use these to 'interpret' experiences and that therefore all new learning is interpreted this way. He refers to this as the 'baggage' that adults bring to learning. In order to be able to learn effectively in different clinical situations we need to recognise how we as individuals engage in learning. This is important for us because we learn most successfully from situations that match our learning style.

There are many ways of explaining how we learn. One that is used commonly is Kolb's learning style inventory (1984). What Kolb suggests is that we fall into the category of one 'style' of learner: those who like to be involved in their own learning and take risks (the Activist); those who value insight and learn by listening and sharing (Reflector); those who think strategically and like factual information (Pragmatist); and those who learn by thinking ideas through (Theorist).

If we understand how we learn, the theory is that we can then select strategies that suit our learning style and be more successful at learning. However, a better strategy might be to acknowledge the learning situations we find useful and those we aren't comfortable with in order to develop in our 'weak' areas and thus become a more 'rounded' learner who can make the most of any learning situation. As learning about nursing occurs in very different situations being an **eclectic** learner is probably a good strategy.

Keywords

Eclectic
Choosing what suits you from a range of different approaches.

There are other ways of explaining our learning styles. Some of you will prefer to start preparing and writing an essay, for example, with an introduction, move on to Chapter 1, Chapter 2 and so on until the conclusion, a very logical, step-by-step approach. Others won't be able to even start writing until they see the 'whole' picture, a 'messy' style of learning where you might start writing parts of chapters first, gradually building up a complete picture. What we have described are 'serialist' and 'holistic' learners. Both strategies have their strengths and weaknesses, with some students able to use both strategies, choosing the one that suits the situation best.

What might be a more important way of looking at learning is to describe our approaches to learning – deep and surface approaches (Entwistle and Tait 1994). If we apply these approaches to reading, for example, the deep approach is where the student 'engages' with the reading, trying to understand and relating the reading to their own experiences. On the other hand, using the surface approach the learner tries to remember what they are reading, with an expectation of having to repeat the information when asked questions. What we need qualified nurses to do is engage in the same way in the care environment, asking questions and trying to understand the situation they find themselves in.

Making sense of nursing care is not easy, no matter what kind of learner you are. In current preregistration nursing programmes 50% of the programme is delivered in clinical practice areas, giving you an opportunity to learn in the 'real situation'. This is where the theory you have learned becomes 'meaningful'. Indeed, when considering learning skills for practice, Spencer (2003) suggests that skills can only be 'learned as an integrated whole' in the clinical environment. This is one example of why the learning that takes place in practice is so important. We have already identified that learning in practice is not easy, because of its intricacy and fast-changing pace.

We have also discussed the importance of reflection if we are to understand the real world of care, as it enables us to 'uncover' the 'complexity of nursing care' (Johns 1995). Reflection uses as its starting point our personal experiences and acknowledges the sense we make of them to create 'new' knowledge. Kolb (1984) describes this as 'experiential learning' and has put together a **model** to help us undertake and understand this. It outlines a series of stages to be gone through but stresses the need to see the process of learning from practice as ongoing, as, having generated and then applied this new knowledge/theory to practice, we then need to consider how effective this was: whether it worked. We need to then go through the process again. This will help 'deepen' our knowledge and understanding.

These stages are identified in Figure 2.1.

⚷ Keywords

Model
A way of representing ideas or theories to help us make sense of them.

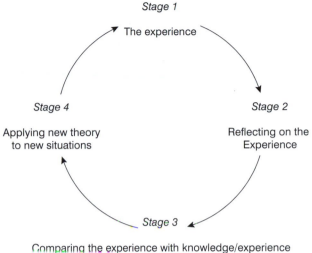

Stage 1
The experience

Stage 4
Applying new theory
to new situations

Stage 2
Reflecting on the
Experience

Stage 3
Comparing the experience with knowledge/experience
Generating new theory

Figure 2.1 *A version of Kolb's learning cycle.*

Social learning theory

Kolb (1984) suggests that this process of experiential learning promotes learning in practice and uses professional experience. Reviewing your practice in this way enables you to deliver care that is of high quality by closing the theory–practice gap and by using appropriate theory to underpin your actions. However, another principle that emerges from this process is the importance of the environment in this learning, in this case the clinical environment. This is described in many education textbooks as 'social learning theory' and has particular relevance for students of nursing. For example, the clinical environment can offer opportunities for the student nurse to learn how to communicate with anxious or confused patients.

This theory, which is mainly credited to Bandura (1977), describes the relationship between the learner and their environment, particularly the importance of observing the actions of others. One of the most powerful ways that student nurses learn is by observing how other nurses deliver care; this enables the student to acquire quite complex patterns of behaviour. However, even when an experienced nurse exhibits behaviours and values, there is no guarantee that the student observer will adopt those behaviours and values. This will depend on how these behaviours are perceived by others, peer approval being an important part of the process.

Student nurses must be allocated a mentor in clinical practice who will take responsibility for teaching and assessing the student.

As well as having a mentor, students often identify, without even realising it, a nurse to 'copy', one who portrays for that student behaviours that they feel reflect the way a 'good' nurse should perform. What influences this choice is probably that this 'good' nurse shares similar beliefs and values, particularly in relation to interpersonal skills such as empathy and sensitivity. These 'role models' can be very powerful in shaping the way student nurses behave. New learners are not always selective. The quality of those who provide a role model will dictate the quality of the nurses produced (Theobald 1995). However, this seems to imply that nursing activities and behaviours, even complex ones, can be learned by observing the 'expert' nurse. There is a process involved, which involves interaction between the student and the environment and the student's motivation. There is therefore a need for the role model to acknowledge this kind of learning and be able to 'step back', enabling the student to participate and then providing feedback.

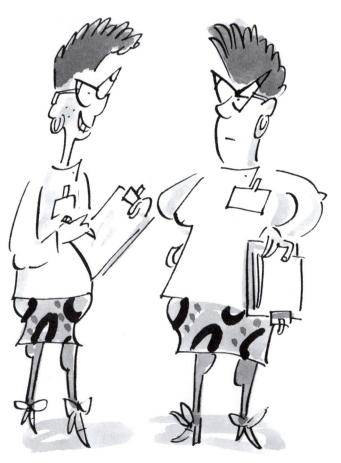

Role modelling is not just about imitation.

The role model then becomes more of a facilitator, encouraging the student to reflect upon and take responsibility for their own learning.

Other authors describe this as 'situated learning theory'. Vygotsky (1978) explains this as the learning that occurs 'through interaction and cooperation with other people in the natural work environment'. It is based upon using an experienced practitioner to guide and take responsibility for the new student. This is often described as the 'apprenticeship' model, as it conjures up a picture of the novice learning from the expert. It provides the new learner with opportunities for imitation, practice, discussion and an element of challenging established beliefs to formulate 'shared' understandings with their colleagues, reinforcing the social nature of learning.

This theory also reinforces the importance of the student being active in the environment, which encourages a sense of 'belonging' and motivation. Fundamental to this theory is the belief that knowledge cannot be separated from the activity, context and culture of the clinical environment.

Our reason for exploring the learning process, focusing on your personal learning and looking at a range of learning strategies, is that we hope to enable you to see yourself as the key to your own learning. This will enable you to develop skills that will allow you to learn in any new situation, by actively considering aspects of your practice that could be changed. This should result in improved practice, with benefits for nursing care and patients. The relating of new knowledge to practice should also help to develop problem-solving and decision-making skills and should help to build your self-confidence. If you are successful in this way it will encourage you to be involved in ongoing reflection and review, ultimately contributing to your continued personal and professional development – lifelong learning. This concept of lifelong learning is revisited in Chapter 6.

Evolving bodies of knowledge

Effken (2000) describes how experienced nurses can respond to individual patients' physical needs using the example of giving an injection. For example, this involves assessing the patient's tissue characteristics – is the patient obese or emaciated, tense or relaxed? – and translating this into a judgement about the amount and direction of force to apply to the syringe and needle. The nurse is using experience to influence the way they carry out an intervention, instinctively making decisions in response to their observation of the patient. These skills when effortless would often be described by the nurse involved as using intuition.

Hansten and Washburn (2000) define intuition as a 'clinical sensing'. They go on to state that this clinical sensing, although not always based on convincing evidence, is based on a sound knowledge base and experience. Schraeder and Fischer (1987) suggest that, when nurses use this knowledge and experience, they can anticipate patient responses instead of having to guess what they might be. Intuition is the 'way of thinking' that develops when knowledge, experience and skills 'come together' (Benner and Tanner 1987).

Cioffi (1997) suggests that intuitive knowing helps nurses see and understand the 'whole' situation rather than the need for a 'staged' and purposeful scrutiny of separate pieces of information, which is how the novice performs. This intuition increases with experience as, the more developed the knowledge base becomes, the easier it becomes for the nurse to skilfully interpret the clinical situation. In other words, because of previous experience the nurse is able to identify even slight clinical changes (Benner and Tanner 1987).

We hope that becoming 'intuitive' will develop your confidence, as confidence is based on your ability, reflecting your coping strategies, evolving problem-solving techniques and communication skills, which will ultimately help you to become skilled and professional practitioners (Dunn and Hansford 2000).

Learning skills for practice

This chapter has attempted to explain to you some of the ways in which we as individuals learn, and the 'thinking' skills we need to develop in order both to underpin safe and competent practice and to improve. It is important that you move from thinking about the development of clinical skills as requiring only repetition (Beeson and Kring 1999) in order to deliver care that is effective and sensitive to patients' needs.

For example, using the measurement of blood pressure as one of the clinical skills that we encounter frequently in practice, we can 'unpack' that skill to look at what we refer to in this book as 'concepts fundamental to all skills delivery', such as risk management and documentation. If we then add the 'professional' thinking skills that we have talked about in this chapter, where all these intersect provides a clear picture of what we mean when we talk about skills for practice, as we firmly believe that these things are inseparable.

We have identified this in the Venn diagram in Figure 2.2.

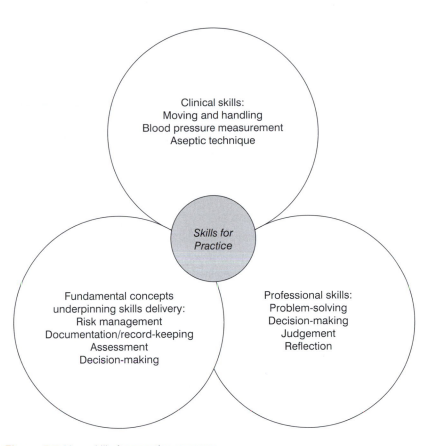

Figure 2.2 *How skills for practice emerge.*

The next chapter will explore those fundamental concepts underpinning all skills delivery.

RRRRRRapid recap

Check your progress so far by working through each of the following questions.

1. What is different about our approach to skill development?

2. Why do we need to alter the way we carry out skills?

3. Why is it important for nurses to use reflection?

4. What 'thinking skills' do nurses use to make sense of patient care needs?

5. How will you identify what helps *you* learn effectively?

If you have difficulty with more than one of the questions, read through the section again to refresh your understanding before moving on.

References

Antrobus, S. (1997) An analysis of nursing in context: the effects of current health policy. *Journal of Advanced Nursing*, **25**, 447–453.

Bandura, A. (1977) *Social Learning Theory*. Prentice-Hall, Englewood Cliffs, NJ.

Beeson, S. and Kring, D.L. (1999) The effects of two teaching methods on nursing students' factual knowledge and performance of psychomotor skills. *Journal of Nursing Education*, **38**, 357–359.

Benner, P. (1984) *From Novice to Expert: Excellence and power in clinical nursing practice*. Addison-Wesley, Menlo Park, CA.

Benner, P. and Tanner, C. (1987) Clinical judgement: how expert nurses use intuition. *American Journal of Nursing*, **87**, 23–31.

Benner, P., Tanner, C. and Chesla, C. (1996) *Experience in Nursing Practice: Caring, clinical judgement and ethics*. Springer, New York.

Boud, D., Keogh, R. and Walker, D. (1985) *Reflection: Turning experience into learning*. Kogan Page, London.

Brookfield, S. (1987) *Developing Critical Thinkers*. Jossey Bass, San Francisco, CA.

Brookfield, S.D. (1995) *Becoming a Critically Reflective Teacher*. Jossey Bass, San Francisco, CA.

Brookfield, S.D. (2000) The concept of critically reflective practice. In: Wilson, A.L. and Hayes, E.R. (eds) *Handbook of Adult and Continuing Education*. Jossey Bass, San Francisco, CA, pp. 110–126.

Chandler, S.M. (2000) Conversation as a way of knowing (doctoral dissertation, University of Colorado at Denver). *Dissertation Abstracts International*, 61, 1726.

Cioffi, J. (1997) Heuristics, servants to intuition, in clinical decision making *Journal of Advanced Nursing*, **26**, 203–208.

Dewey, J. (1933) *How We Think: A restatement of the relation of reflective thinking to the educative process*, 2nd edn. Heath & Co., New York.

Dreyfus, S. and Dreyfus, H. (1980) cited in Benner, P. (1984) *From Novice to Expert: Excellence and power in clinical nursing practice*. Addison-Wesley, Menlo Park, CA.

Dunn, S.V. and Hansford, B. (2000) Undergraduate nursing students' perceptions of their clinical learning environment. *Journal of Advanced Nursing*, **25**, 1299–1306.

Effken, J. (2000) Informational basis for expert tuition. *Journal of Advanced Nursing*, **34**, 246–255.

Entwistle, N.J. and Tait, H. (1994) *The Revised Approaches to Studying Inventory*. Centre for Research into Learning and Instruction, University of Edinburgh, Edinburgh.

Gibbs, G. (1988) *Learning by Doing: A guide to teaching and learning methods*. Further Education Unit, Oxford Polytechnic, Oxford.

Glaze, J.E. (2002) Stages in coming to terms with reflection: student advanced nurse practitioners perceptions of their reflective journeys. *Journal of Advanced Nursing*, **37**, 265–272.

Hansten, R. and Washburn, M. (2000) Intuition in professional practice: executive and staff perceptions. *The Journal of Nursing Administration*, **30**, 185–189.

Johns, C. (1995) The value of reflective practice for nursing. *Journal of Clinical Nursing*, **4**, 23–30.

Kolb, D. (1984) *Experiential Learning: Experiences as a source of learning and development*. Prentice-Hall, Englewood Cliffs, NJ.

Mezirow, J. (1990) *Fostering Critical Reflection in Adulthood: A guide to transformative and emancipatory learning*. Jossey Bass, San Francisco, CA.

Mezirow, J. (1991) *Transformative Dimensions of Adult Learning*. Jossey Bass, San Francisco, CA.

Miller, M.A. (1992) Outcomes evaluation: measuring critical thinking. *Journal of Advanced Nursing*, **17**, 1401–1407.

Paul, R. (1992) *Critical Thinking: What every person needs to survive in a rapidly changing world*, 2nd edn. Foundation for Critical Thinking, Santa Rosa, CA.

Price, B. (2004) Demonstrating critical thought. *Nursing Standard* **18**(18), 32.

Ruth-Sahd, L.A. (2003) Reflective practice: a critical analysis of data-based studies and implications for nursing education. *Journal of Nursing Education*, **42**, 488.

Schon, D. (1983) *The Reflective Practitioner: How professionals think in action*. Basic Books, London.

Schraeder, B. and Fischer, D. (1987) Using intuitive knowledge in the neonatal intensive care nursery. *Holistic Nursing Practice*, **1**, 45–51.

Spencer, J. (2003) Learning and teaching in the clinical environment *British Medical Journal*, **326**, 591–595.

Theobald, M. (1995) Nursing must first become a profession of graduates. *British Journal of Nursing*, **5**, 0–7.

Vygotsky, L.S. (1978) *Mind in Society*. Harvard University Press, Cambridge, MA.

Wilkinson, J.M. (1992) *Nursing Process in Action: A critical thinking approach*. Addison-Wesley, Redwood City, CA.

Further reading

Jasper, M. (2003) *Beginning Reflective Practice*. Nelson Thornes, Cheltenham.

3

Key concepts underpinning all skill delivery

Learning outcomes

By the end of this chapter you should be able to:

- Outline the key concepts underpinning all skill delivery
- Identify your values and beliefs about nursing
- Be aware of some of your attitudes and prejudices.

This chapter will not tell you how to assess, as there are many other sources of information that will do that; what this chapter will do is to take you a stage further in fostering the model of skill development that was introduced to you in Chapters 1 and 2. This is a very long chapter but we make no apologies for that, as it is an important chapter because it introduces you to what we consider are the fundamental concepts that are the basis of all skill delivery for nurses and other health care professionals. In keeping with the rest of the chapters in this book, there are reflective exercises and case studies that will stimulate your learning and development. The reflective exercises contained in this chapter will help you to clarify your values and beliefs about nursing, become more aware of your personal qualities and begin to identify your attitudes and prejudices. A case study will provide you, a novice practitioner, with a benchmark for expert practice.

Setting the scene

Traditionally, nurses have used procedure books/manuals and nursing care texts in order to identify a how-to-do-it recipe for clinical skills. In our interactions with both clinical staff and students it often appears that many people seem to work with the mindset that clinical skills will develop just by working in clinical areas. To us this process seems to be akin to the process of osmosis – just by being there and doing, not only will you absorb the ability to practise competently but you will also develop your practice to become what Benner (1984) calls an 'expert practitioner'. Oh, that it was that easy! Unfortunately there is no easy way. Clinical skills need to be worked at, first to gain competence and then to gain mastery.

As we said in the previous chapter, you will naturally be very focused around the 'how to' at the beginning of your programme. For example, when performing a wound dressing your concerns will be with:

- Have I got all of the equipment I need?
- What is sterile and what is not?
- What can I touch?
- How do I manipulate the equipment?

As you become more practised in this skill you should then progress to considering such things as:

- What does the patient feel about this procedure? In other words, what do I notice about the patient's behaviour, e.g. are they displaying any signs of anxiety?
- What is the patient saying to me about how they feel about having the procedure performed?
- What does the patient say we are going to do to him/her?
- What's the most comfortable position for the patient?
- Will the procedure be painful – if so what analgesic can I give beforehand and what time should I give it in order to give it time to work?
- Do I need to give the patient specific advice and/or information?
- What's happening in the patient's life that may be impacting on him/her?
- How does the patient feel about his/her health problem?
- Are there any guidelines, national or local about the care of patients like this?
- How is this nursing care to be recorded?
- Is there evidence of wound healing?
- Have the factors that affect wound healing been considered, e.g. nutritional status?

Inherent in this example of performing a wound dressing is the complexity of everyday practice. In the beginning it will be difficult for you to be able to see the wood for the trees. However, you need to be aware that professional practice needs time and experience to acquire. This book will clarify how you can learn to develop as an expert professional. Throughout this chapter we are going to equip you with a broader understanding of this process that will take you beyond the recipe stage.

In order to support the unfolding of your practice skills this chapter will identify and explore the intricate skills that you need in order to become a competent practitioner. Throughout the chapter our unique approach to clinical skill development will help to identify how you can master these skills. As you will see when you read further into this chapter, the skills that we believe are key to becoming an expert practitioner include:

- Assessment
- Communication
- Professional judgement and decision-making
- Risk management
- Record keeping and documentation, and
- Managing uncertainty.

These skills we have called 'enablers', as these are the fundamental skills that provide the means for expert professional practice. However, there are other skills that you will need to learn, which will ensure that you develop the 'enabling' skills. These are the 'softer' skills and are to do with the 'personal' and the 'self'. The skills related to the Personal include:

- Personal qualities
- Social skills and
- Cultural awareness,

whereas the skills to do with the Self include:

- Emotional intelligence and
- Emotional labour.

It is important that you recognise that these are not isolated skills but see them as interacting, and appreciate that developing these skills will help you to reach the peak of your personal abilities or, as Maslow (1987) puts it, reach 'self-actualisation'. In order to practise as an expert nurse you will need to learn to bring together and hone your personal qualities, personal philosophies and cultural awareness with your propositional knowledge and understanding and moral stance. It is the ability to develop and use all these skills that sets apart the expert nurse from the advanced beginner.

While Benner (1984) documents the route that nurses take when they move from 'novice to expert', her work only describes what the results of the journey are. She gives no help or advice in her study that shows you how to become an expert nurse. Her work only identifies the distinguishing features of expert nurses. If you consider the career pathway of a qualified nurse as a continuum, then a student nurse at the start of his/her programme would be on one end of the continuum and the expert practitioner would be at the other end. Sadly, you do not automatically become an expert practitioner after having served a certain number of years. You can deliver patient care on a daily basis for 40 years and still function as what Dreyfus and Dreyfus (in Benner 1984) call an 'advanced beginner'. In order to develop your clinical practice to the extent that you become an expert practitioner you need to be able to recognise that the process is one of skill development. Consequently, you need not only to be aware of this process but also how you are going to become engaged in it.

Assessment

Assessment is, we believe, one of the key concepts that underpin all nursing practice. The assessment process is intricate, dynamic and continuous and includes a number of higher-order skills that you will need to learn. As assessment is a complex skill it takes beginning nurses a number of years to fully develop their assessment skills. This is because you need a combination of knowledge, skills and experience. Like all complex skills, assessment is a difficult skill to learn and there would seem to be three main reasons for this.

Tacit knowledge

First, many skilled nurses find it difficult to clearly describe their thinking processes (Luker and Kenrick 1992, Meerabeau 1992, MacLeod 1996, Meyer and Batchup 1997). Consequently, they are unable to explain clearly to you how they have used the patient assessment data to decide which nursing interventions to employ. Meerabeau (1992) suggests that this is because their expert knowledge has been developed over a period of time. To describe the knowledge these practitioners have acquired that they find difficult to articulate, Meerabeau uses the term 'tacit knowledge'. Such 'tacit knowledge' develops, and is refined, each time a nurse is exposed to clinical situations that are very similar. As this integrated knowledge is subtly built up over a period of time it becomes difficult to separate out theoretical knowledge from knowledge gained from experience. Schon (1983) also refers to this process in his seminal work The ***Reflective Practitioner***, when he explores how professionals develop their practice.

This means that you, as a student nurse observing expert nurses, will find it impossible to view their thinking processes and as a result will often find it difficult to see how they have come to the decision(s) that they have. It also means that you need to be exposed to a variety of clinical situations to enable you to build up a repertoire of clinical experiences that you can use in your thinking processes.

Keywords

Reflective practitioner
A practitioner who regularly thinks about their practice. They use this process to examine their actions and understandings to improve their knowledge and skills. In this way the practitioner learns and develops both personally and professionally.

Secondly, like any skill that you learn, the skills underpinning nursing take time to develop, as you need to be able to practise the skills many times in order to become expert. Take an everyday example from life that many of you will have no doubt experienced – learning to drive a car. Like nursing practice, driving a car is a complex skill to learn. First of all you have to master coordinating clutch, accelerator and handbrake in order to pull away. However that's not all you have to do, although that's difficult enough. Not only do you have to be able to steer the car but you also have to be able to accelerate to a safe driving speed to suit both the legal speed limits and the road conditions. Alongside learning to coordinate your feet in tune with the engine speed you have to look not at what your feet are doing but at the road ahead, the road behind you and to each side of you before you start to pull away. You also need to be aware of the behaviour of other road users and pedestrians in order to predict possible dangers.

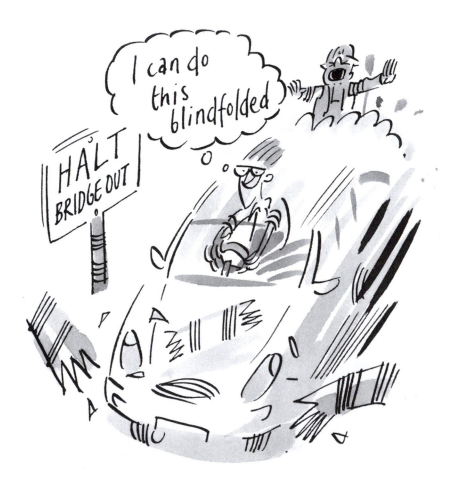

Reflective activity

If you have learned or are learning to drive a car, think back to the very first driving lesson that you had. If you haven't ever had a driving lesson, ask someone you know who has.

- During your first lesson how many times did you stall or nearly stall the car you were driving before you could pull away smoothly each time?
- What was it that you did that helped you overcome this difficulty?

No wonder that when we are learning to drive a car we feel as though we have two left feet and that there is information overload. We, the authors, would argue that learning to nurse in today's NHS is even more complex than learning to drive a car. When you are learning to drive there is an instructor with you watching and analysing your performance, followed by a discussion and guidance that is aimed at improving your performance. However, as a student nurse there will not be an instructor with you every inch of the way until you are deemed qualified to nurse. Which brings us to the third reason why clinical skills are difficult to learn.

This is because in many of the clinical situations you find yourself in you will be working with little direct supervision. This is no fault of your mentor. This is because many NHS institutions do not appear to have the qualified staff to directly supervise student nurses all the time. Alongside this, student nurse learning is increasingly expected to be self-directed and this applies more and more to clinical practice as well as academic learning. This concept of self-direction appears to be contrary to the established literature on skills learning (de Tornyay 1971, Bandura 1986, Lave and Wenger 1991, Quinn 1995). This literature suggests that students learning a skill should be given the opportunity to observe a skill at least once and then to practise the skill under supervision a number of times. It is also suggested that the mentor should give feedback to the learner during and after carrying out the skill. During this time of supervised practice the mentor will be able to guide the student and then give feedback on the student's performance.

Given that in many clinical situations you will be working without close supervision it will sometimes be difficult for you to analyse your performance and give yourself constructive feedback. You can of course use the patient's comments as feedback. However when you do this you should always consider the following two points that will help to validate this type of feedback: its reliability and validity. If the patient is an expert in their own care then the feedback is

> ## Reflective activity
>
> Consider when either you or someone you know learned to drive. You always had an instructor in the car with you.
>
> - Do you think that learner drivers could be self-directed?
> - Should the level of supervision available to learner drivers be available to learner nurses?
> - How do you think you could validate your performance when you are not being directly supervised?

probably very useful. If the patient is not an expert in their own care then you may find the feedback ego-massaging but it might not be very reliable or valid.

> ## Over to you
>
> Consider how you might validate your performance when not directly supervised.

Yes, reflection on and in action will help you to do this. Remember, in Chapter 2 it was suggested that in order to do this you need to think regularly about particular events that have happened to you in practice and then identify the key concepts involved. Once you have done this you can find the evidence you need to allow you to examine your actions. Your thought processes will enable you then to analyse your actions and responses in light of the evidence:

- Could I have done anything differently? If so what?
- Did I miss any clues?
- Could I have collected any other data?
- Could my communication/interpersonal skills have been improved?
- Did I use all my senses? If not, why not?

Using the process of reflection will improve your clinical problem solving abilities (Jasper 2003).

As we said earlier, assessment is a fundamental skill to learn. However, it's not only us who feel that assessment is a key skill. The **Quality Assurance Agency for Higher Education** (2001) has stated that those qualifying as nurses, regardless of branch, should be able to perform a systematic assessment of a client and then use this information to produce a documented nursing management plan. Patient assessment is therefore a vital aspect of nursing care,

Keywords

Quality Assurance Agency for Higher Education

The agency charged by the government with ensuring that the programmes/courses offered by universities in the UK reach a required standard.

⚷ Keywords

Nursing interventions
The activities that nurses use to deliver nursing care to patients.

as it allows the nurse to plan **nursing interventions**. During a patient assessment you will need both to gather information about the patient and to make judgements about what might be complex and diverse assessment data in order to plan patient care. Critical thinking and decision-making are therefore just two of the essential skills involved in producing a complete and accurate assessment.

It is difficult either to describe a standard assessment or to produce a protocol for a patient assessment because nurses are caring for people (well and sick) in a variety of environments. In any 24 hours in today's NHS there will be patients in need of either urgent or non-urgent care in a variety of health care settings. These include outpatient clinics, day surgery units, intensive care units, NHS Direct and nursing homes. Some patients are critically ill, some patients are 'walking wounded', yet others are well and are being given advice and support about aspects of health promotion. The assessment process, therefore, has to be a system that will meet the needs of all patients and nurses, whichever health care setting they may be in.

Use of models in the assessment process

⚷ Keywords

Biomedical model
The central value of this model is physical health. It recognises that the body is a biochemical and physical system. This model gives less value to the psychological, emotional or social functioning and wellbeing of the individual than to the physical wellbeing.

Psychosocial model
The core value of this model is to consider both the psychological and the social processes that people are involved in and how these can affect health and wellbeing.

Much nursing care is said to be based on the **biomedical model** (Pearson and Vaughan 1991), by which nurses provide physical care for the patient's physical problems, which arise from medical conditions. This model, however, reduces the body to a set of related parts, separates the mind from the body and as a result can fail to recognise the psychosocial and cultural needs of patients. However, you may find that using a nursing model of care that provides a framework for your assessment may be helpful, for example Roper, Logan and Tierney's Activities of Living model (Roper *et al.* 1996). This **psychosocial model**, along with its corruptions and variants, is frequently used as a basis for initial assessment documentation in many hospital wards. However, there are many nursing models available for you to use. We would suggest that you familiarise yourself with the one that you feel most comfortable with – this will be a model that fits in with your values and beliefs. For example, if you believe strongly that individuals are responsible for their own health, then Orem's self-care model (Orem 1996) might be the nursing model you would feel most comfortable using.

Yet many patient groups and some nurses criticise both these nursing models and the medical model (Walsh 1998). They suggest that such models are nursing-focused rather than patient-focused and that nurses should use a more social model of care instead.

If you don't use a model it could be said that the care that you consequently provide is founded on an individual belief system.

It has been suggested (Walsh 1998) that individual nurses working from their own personal belief systems seem to produce indifferent, disjointed and incomplete assessments. Indeed, Sutcliffe (1994) and Robb (1997) go so far as to suggest that continuity of care can be achieved only when those involved share similar nursing philosophies.

Defining your values and beliefs about nursing

Reflective activity

What is your nursing philosophy (the values and beliefs that you hold about nursing)? If you haven't yet given this any thought you really need to begin to clarify it. Here are some questions to ask yourself that will help you to establish your nursing philosophy.

   If this is your first attempt to examine your values and beliefs about nursing then you should do this activity more than once. We are asking you to do something that is difficult so expect it to take you some time. You may have to come back to it a few times. Be honest with yourself. If you're not, then the only person you're fooling is yourself.

- I want to be a qualified nurse because . . .
- I believe that nurses are . . .
- I believe that the aim of nursing is . . .
- As a nurse my practice will be . . .
- I believe that all patients are . . .
- I believe that some patients are . . .
- I believe that all patients' families are . . .
- I believe that all doctors are . . .
- I believe that all health care professionals are . . .
- My beliefs about health are . . .
- Being healthy to me is . . .

Patient diversity

The people who are our patients not only come from diverse cultural and socioeconomic backgrounds but they also may have a variety of health care problems. Many people have chronic physical diseases while others are having an acute episode of physical ill health. Some will also have mental health problems and others may also have a learning disability. Our patients will also have had a wide variety of life experiences so as a result each patient is a unique individual. Assessment is needed, therefore, to reflect the needs of individual patients and their families. Indeed Walsh (1998) goes as far as suggesting that without a comprehensive assessment, nursing care is

⊶┳ *Keywords*

Systematic assessment

An assessment that is orderly and methodical in the way it is carried out. This usually means following a model, e.g. the Activities of Living model or a systems based model. However, if using a systems based model you must remember to add psychosocial aspects to your assessment tool.

Continuous assessment

An assessment that is ongoing during the whole of the patient's involvement with the care system.

routinised and 'impersonal'. In order to be comprehensive the **assessment** should be both **systematic** and **continuous**.

Reflective activity

A skill is an activity that we learn to do. It is something that we learn through practice and reflection. In order to develop your skills you need to have a number of personal qualities. These qualities include:

- Commitment
- Determination
- Motivation
- Perseverance
- Positive thinking
- Self-awareness

Which of these qualities do you believe that you have? If you don't have all of them, consider how you are going to acquire them. Aspects of your preregistration course should help you acquire some of these qualities, e.g. self-awareness.

Learning a skill

Over to you

Identify two skills that you can perform well. How did you learn those skills?

Write a list of the components that make up the two skills you have just identified.

We, the authors, all learned to catheterise female patients. What we learned to do was to bring together all the following skills and their underpinning knowledge and understanding: information giving, active listening, answering questions, gaining consent, maintaining privacy and dignity, preventing infection, aseptic technique, passing a urethral catheter, maintenance of urine drainage, safe disposal of waste, monitoring intake and output, anatomy and physiology of the urinary tract, disordered physiology, bacteriology.

The way we often learn skills is by breaking them into their component parts and learning how to do each part and then linking all the parts together. So, what we will consider next are the component skills of gathering and interpreting clinical information, or in other words the constituent parts of assessment.

Skills of assessment

In order to carry out a successful assessment you will need to use a combination of all the following skills:

- Data collection
  - Observation
  - Measuring
  - Interviewing
- Communication
- Record keeping and documentation
- Risk management
- Professional judgement and decision-making
- Managing uncertainty.

The assessment process can be defined as the gathering and analysis of information about a specific patient that allows you to determine patient problems. If you would like to use a more contemporary term than gathering information you can think of assessment as data collection and analysis.

Data collection

Assessment consists of a number of the processes described above, which, although they are described individually, are often carried out simultaneously. An assessment should be both valid and reliable. In other words, an assessment must assess what it claims to assess and produce the same result regardless of which nurse performs it. Regardless of the way that it is carried out, the assessment will rely on the nurse gathering information about the patient.

The data that you collect will be either small or large amounts of information that you can see, hear or smell, or that the patient/carer can tell you about. For example, it could be that when you are with Mr Ferry, a patient who has had a stroke, you can see that his lips are very dry and cracked. You may also notice that he is having difficulty swallowing. When you question Mr Ferry he complains of thirst. This would therefore lead you to find out when Mr Ferry last drank any fluid. You would also need to ascertain what kind of fluid it was that he drank and how much he drank. At the same time you notice whether he has poor skin turgor (loss of the normal elasticity of the skin). Then you will need to ask yourself what all this information means. It could be that this patient is dehydrated. If this is the case then further assessment information will need to be gathered to confirm your conclusions.

We have found that it is useful to ask yourself the following question:

- Can I organise any of the information that I'm collecting into a pattern?

We think it will help if you think of assessment as being like a seesaw.

When you sit on one side of a seesaw you need to have someone on the other end to act as a counterbalance. Otherwise the seesaw is out of balance and doesn't work. The seesaw itself balances on a fulcrum (pivot).

When we apply the analogy of a seesaw to assessment, on a seat on one end of the seesaw are the holistic fundamental skills such as empathy, active listening, trust, presence and what Radwin (1996) has called 'knowing the patient', while on the other seat on the other end are the specific skills like observation, measurement and medicine administration. Holding these two ends in balance by acting as a fulcrum are the contextual issues such as patient concerns (e.g. pain, role change or financial difficulties) or resources (e.g. an extremely obese man is to be admitted to a hospital ward and there is no available bed or hoist that he will fit into).

When using this model, visualise which end of the seesaw your information will sit on. When you have considered this think about what contextual issues the seesaw seats are balancing on. For example, if you consider the scenario of Mr Ferry mentioned earlier, then on one side of the seesaw there are the holistic skills of active listening and empathy while on the other side are the observing and questioning skills. These skills are balancing on: the patient's anxieties (his father had a stroke at the same age and his father died 2 weeks after his stroke); the National Clinical Guidelines for Stroke (Royal College of Physicians 2002); and today's staff shortage (two members of staff rang in sick this morning).

This will help you to translate the data that you collect so that you can see what all this information is telling you. It may also suggest to you what other data you should be looking for. However, always be careful not to reach conclusions too early. One piece of information on its own can often be misleading. Remember that you should always be trying to balance the seesaw, which is the holistic skills on one seat, the specific skills on the other and the contextual issues as the fulcrum. In the case of Mr Ferry the data could be telling you that this patient is dehydrated because he is unable to lift a cup to drink from, he may not be able to swallow properly, or he is so anxious that he has forgotten to drink anything. This may have been compounded by the lack of staff available to assist him.

Often, large amounts of information will be available. However, you will have to learn to use your knowledge, skills and experience to decide which information is significant. Because of this, the assessment outcomes of individual nurses can and do differ. This is

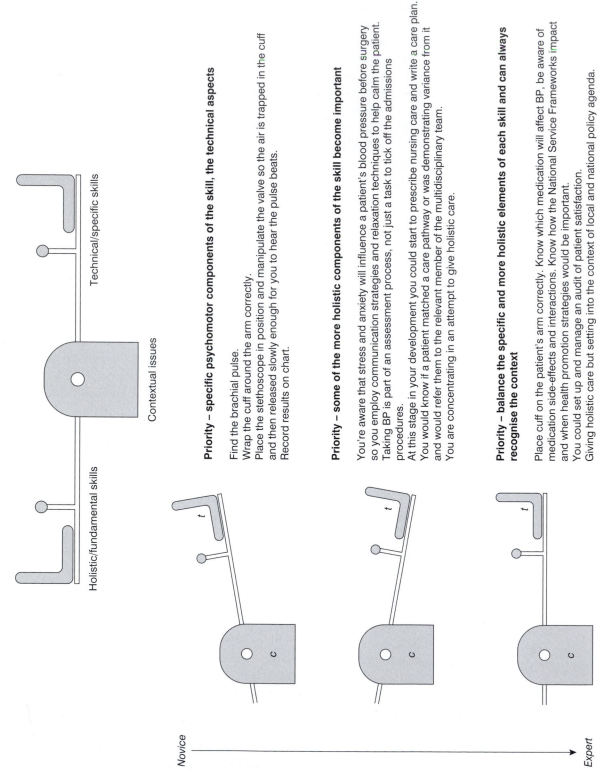

Technical/specific skills

Contextual issues

Holistic/fundamental skills

Priority – specific psychomotor components of the skill, the technical aspects

Find the brachial pulse.
Wrap the cuff around the arm correctly.
Place the stethoscope in position and manipulate the valve so the air is trapped in the cuff and then released slowly enough for you to hear the pulse beats.
Record results on chart.

Priority – some of the more holistic components of the skill become important

You're aware that stress and anxiety will influence a patient's blood pressure before surgery so you employ communication strategies and relaxation techniques to help calm the patient. Taking BP is part of an assessment process, not just a task to tick off the admissions procedures.
At this stage in your development you could start to prescribe nursing care and write a care plan. You would know if a patient matched a care pathway or was demonstrating variance from it and would refer them to the relevant member of the multidisciplinary team.
You are concentrating in an attempt to give holistic care.

Priority – balance the specific and more holistic elements of each skill and can always recognise the context

Place cuff on the patient's arm correctly. Know which medication will affect BP, be aware of medication side-effects and interactions. Know how the National Service Frameworks impact and when health promotion strategies would be important.
You could set up and manage an audit of patient satisfaction.
Giving holistic care but setting into the context of local and national policy agenda.

Novice

Expert

Figure 3.1 *The seesaw effect – assessing blood pressure.*

because personal experiences and how they are rationalised influence nurses as well as patients. Nurses are not like computers with uniform data-handling techniques; they are people and as such they interpret things in different ways. They are influenced by a whole compendium of knowledge, experiences, prejudices and attitudes unique to each of them.

Over to you

In order to practise in an anti-discriminatory manner you need to be self-aware.

- Do you know what your attitudes and prejudices are? It will help you towards working in an anti-discriminatory manner if you do know what your prejudices and attitudes are, so spend 5 minutes writing a list.
- Have you identified any attitudes that you need to work on to ensure that you practise in a non-discriminatory fashion?
- If you have identified some then congratulate yourself for being honest. Many of us have attitudes that are developed mostly through fear and lack of understanding. We need to acknowledge them and work to ensure that we develop an understanding of why we have those attitudes.

Communication

During any assessment you will be applying a variety of communication skills so that you can collect accurate and meaningful data. Interviewing is a key requisite. You will also have to bear in mind that if the assessment is part of the admission process then this will be the first stage in developing a therapeutic relationship with the patient/carer and their family. So you will need to consider how you will apply the communication skills that you will learn during your course. Give consideration to the following:

- Venue – where will the interview take place? Is there sufficient privacy and comfort? If not, how can you strive to ensure that there is?
- What about seating provision? Where are you going to sit in relation to the patient/carer? Consider using **SOLER** (Egan 2002)
- Time considerations
- Interviewing – types of questions – open (encourage a wordy answer) or closed (can be answered with one word). For example, it would be appropriate to ask closed questions of someone who is very breathless or who finds it difficult to speak for whatever reason. However you will need to remember that closed questions

🔑 Keywords

SOLER

S – sitting
O – open
L – leaning forward
E – eye contact
R – relaxed

produce very limited responses so questions will have to be constructed carefully

- Active listening
- Being non-judgemental
- Being aware of both different abilities and disabling environments
- Being aware of different cultures
- Appropriate language.

While carrying out an assessment you should also bear in mind that, for some people that you will care for, their bodies and minds are no longer under their voluntary control. This could also obscure the assessment process. When a person's body or mind, or possibly both, is no longer under their wilful control, this can present you with considerable difficulties when making any assessment. This is particularly so if you have only recently come into contact with this person. At times like this you should consider that it might be helpful to have the next of kin or other such person to assist with the assessment. Remember that, whenever possible, the patient should give their consent to this.

Verbal and non-verbal communication may no longer relate to expressions of need and can be open to misinterpretation. The removal of clothing, for example, could have sexual connotations or simply mean that the individual is feeling hot, or that their clothing is in some way uncomfortable. Also, an individual's ability or inability to perform Activities of Living (Roper *et al.* 1996) may be influenced by external factors such as the staff on duty, the time of day and the presence or absence of a particular relative.

You also need to remember that some patients may be unwilling or unable to contribute to the assessment process, for a variety of reasons. It may be that the patient doesn't understand why you are collecting all this information, they may be in too much pain (either physical or emotional) to make any kind of contribution or they may be too embarrassed. It requires sensitivity on your part to be aware of these cues.

For example, 'At any one time one adult in six suffers from one or other form of mental illness. In other words mental illness is as common as asthma' (Department of Health 1999). Consequently, many of the patients you will care for will be experiencing a mental illness as well as the physical disease. Therefore you should ensure you explore your patient's **cognition**, **affect** and behaviour. Remember, how they think will affect how they feel, and how they feel will affect how they think; this will have an impact on their behaviour.

Keywords

Cognition
A person's comprehension of who they are, where they are and what's happening to them, and their ability to think and reason.

Affect
The way someone feels.

In theory, all assessments should be holistic to provide nursing care to the whole person. However, in reality there may be times when this is not possible. Such times will be when the patient's life is threatened by their condition, e.g. airway obstruction. The focus of the assessment at such times is to collect enough data to make a diagnosis and instigate immediate life-saving strategies. The holistic assessment will come later once the patient is out of danger. However, this is not to say that the care given will not be humanistic: for example, the patient's privacy and dignity should be protected at all times, even during life-threatening situations.

With a patient assessment the amount of information you need to collect will depend on why you are doing the assessment. For example, a wound assessment will be much more straightforward than a moving and handling assessment of a patient with a dense right-sided hemiplegia (paralysis of the right side of the body) following a cerebrovascular accident (CVA or stroke).

Professional judgement and decision-making

During a patient assessment you will need to both gather information about the patient and make judgements about what might be complex and diverse assessment data in order to plan patient care. Professional judgement and decision-making are therefore just two of the essential skills involved in producing a complete and accurate assessment. They are also fundamental to care planning and to the evaluation of care. Essential in this process of making decisions is clinical reasoning. Clinical reasoning is where you collect and interpret the information that you find during your assessment. It could include what you see, what the patient tells you and how the patient is behaving, or it could be gathered from other sources such as measurement of vital signs or blood values. You will then think about the information that you have and whether this is similar to anything that you know about. As your experience grows and your knowledge and understanding deepens, this becomes a process that you are often not fully conscious of.

Integrating different aspects of information about a situation, person or object that allow us to reach an overall conclusion is said to be the process of judgement (Maule 2001). The following example demonstrates how a novice and an expert analyse the information that they collect and make a professional judgement in the light of that information.

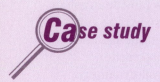

Case study

Judgement of a novice and an expert practitioner

Novice practitioner

The student nurse inspects a clean, stitched wound that is red, so she thinks that the wound is infected. She has come to this conclusion because she knows that redness is a sign of infection.

However, compare this with the wound assessment thought processes of an expert practitioner.

Expert practitioner

This is a clean, stitched wound that looks a little swollen and is a little red along the suture line. The patient's pulse and temperature are within normal range. The patient is not complaining unduly of pain. The wound is neither causing the patient any discomfort nor does the patient appear distressed. Therefore the expert practitioner concludes that the wound is healing normally and showing signs of the inflammatory process. The expert knows that inflammation is the body's response to both injury and infection.

In this example differentiation is made between the inflammatory process due to injury and inflammation due to the infective process. The expert practitioner is using the understanding that she has gained from seeing a wide variety of wounds, from normally healing wounds to delayed healing wounds. Alongside these thoughts, this practitioner also applies her knowledge of normal and disordered physiology to interpret the clinical features that she sees. She has also considered the patient and the context of the situation.

This implies that an expert practitioner will be using a wide variety of clinical information in order to make a judgement about a patient's condition. Even if the practitioner is not aware of the process happening, they are using information such as how the patient looks, what are the patient's vital signs, what the patient's medical condition is and how the patient is behaving. Professional judgement and decision-making is about thinking in a logical manner to reach a conclusion or conclusions.

It may be that you are involved in assisting with a patient who has had a life-threatening event, for example cardiac arrest. In situations such as these time is of the essence, so you don't have time to think. Your actions must be automatic. Consequently you follow either the basic life support or advanced life support algorithm laid down by the Resuscitation Council (UK) (2000). In other situations that are not life-threatening you will be thinking and reasoning by exploring the situation from all sides, taking into account a variety of knowledge and understanding. You will be trying to consider all eventualities and explore all possibilities. If you are thinking critically you will be trying to generate ideas that match the situation, not thinking 'We always do this this way'. Your thinking should be guided by three key questions: Why?, How? and When?

This is the process of critical thinking and it is fundamental to good decision-making and evidence-based practice. Critical thinking is the ability to reason and reasoning is fundamental to problem-solving. These skills are essential in exercising professional judgement. Coming to professional judgements based on critical thinking ensures that your clinical decisions are rooted in more than tradition, ritual and guesswork. Like other skills, critical thinking needs practice in order to develop and improve.

When you have made a judgement about the patient's condition you will then have to make a decision about whether any nursing action is necessary and if so what will the intervention be.

Using evidence

In order to make decisions about a patient's nursing care you will have to learn to weigh up the possible intervention(s) and examine these in the light of research that supports or opposes the possible intervention(s). Practising in this way is known as evidence-based practice. Sackett *et al.* (1997, p. 23) suggest that evidence-based practice is 'The conscientious, explicit and judicious use of best evidence in making decisions about the care of individual patients'.

Decision-making has to be informed by evidence. Evidence-based practice is rooted in the practice of medicine and doctors have always considered the gold standard of evidence to be research that uses randomised controlled trials. However, as a nurse you will need to have a wider view of evidence than this. While randomised controlled trials are appropriate forms of evidence in some situations they do not meet the requirements for all that is nursing. As nurses we must use evidence from a wider range of research philosophies. This will mean using research from the qualitative end of the research continuum, such as ethnographies, case studies or action research. Rigorous qualitative studies with an in-depth analysis of data and a focus on examining alternative explanations will also help us to better understand patients' experiences, attitudes and beliefs.

Accountability

Nurses working in health care in the UK are accountable for their practice and ultimately for the decisions that they take (Nursing and Midwifery Council 2002).

Society today expects appropriate, effective, efficient, timely and affordable care from nurses in whichever context they practise. Therefore qualified nurses should base their decision-making and consequent interventions on the best available evidence.

Managing uncertainty

However, nursing is a relatively new and emerging profession and as a result it has a limited research base. Consequently this will often present you with a dilemma, as there are times when there is either inadequate evidence or even no evidence at all to support your decision-making. All nurses face this difficulty from time to time but there are two important things to be learned from this. The first difficulty that needs to be addressed is how to make a decision without sound reliable and valid evidence and the second difficulty really poses you a challenge. If there isn't sufficient evidence to support a nursing intervention, this identifies areas of practice that need research. So, as it was you who needed the evidence and it wasn't there, consider if it should be you who initiates the research.

Another difficulty that many nurses often have is that in many situations the outcomes of care are uncertain. The reason for this is as nurses we deal with human beings and, as you are aware, each person is different both in personality and life experiences, as well as physically, socially and emotionally. Consequently, how each person reacts to illness and to health education is different. Therefore it isn't always possible to predict the outcomes of nursing care or medical treatment.

Two metaphors that are often used by clinicians to describe their daily work are juggling and swimming like a swan. If you examine both of these metaphors in more detail you will begin to see how complicated the process of decision-making and professional judgement is. Juggling, or keeping all the balls in the air at once, can be described as an unstable environment made stable by the balancing abilities of the artist. Expert nurses frequently make unstable environments stable by their decision-making and judgement skills and, like swans, they appear on the surface to be swimming calmly and serenely to their goal when if you could look under the water they are frantically paddling as hard as they can. Both learning to juggle and learning to swim like a swan takes time, practice and motivation.

One of the important messages to take away from this chapter is that, while external evidence can inform, it is not meant to replace expertise and experience. External evidence is only part of the decision-making process. The other parts involve not only an understanding of the pathophysiology of the disease but also an understanding of the social, cultural and psychological context of the patient's lived experiences. In other words all patients have a life in which their ill health is only a part (Selder 1989, Liaschenko 1998). This is fundamental to holistic, person-centred practice (Watson 1988, Benner and Wrubel 1989, Johns 1994).

Reflective activity

There are three activities that are fundamental to both reflective and evidence-based practice. These are knowing:

- What constitutes reliable and valid evidence
- Where to look for the evidence
- How to critique the evidence.

Think about these three questions and ask yourself if you have all these skills.

If you haven't yet acquired these three key skills consider how you will learn them. Perhaps they will be a useful addition to your personal development planning.

Theory Into Practice

Holistic, person-centred care is more than individualised patient care. Individualised patient care usually means giving patients choice over some aspects of the care such as washing and dressing, food and drink and sleeping. Holistic care has also been termed humanistic care by Watson (1988).

Practising in such a way means identifying and acknowledging the patient's values and beliefs, recognising their coping strategies and noticing subtle changes in their communication patterns and behaviour. It also means perceiving not only feelings that the patient may be experiencing, e.g. embarrassment, but also how these feelings affect the individual patient. Lawler's (1991) research clearly identifies how some nurses know and understand people.

Interpreting and analysing

We consider that the assessment process must take into account the context of patient care. This is particularly important because, as you will notice, patients rarely seem to have problems that are one-dimensional. The majority of patient problems are complex. This means that you can't consider the patient's physical problems in isolation. You will need to consider them in their psychological, environmental, social and cultural context, as well as the physical one.

The following case study will illustrate this.

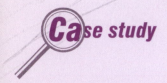

Shonagh – physical problems in their context

Mrs Shonagh Devine is a 36-year-old woman who has been a patient in your ward many times as result of Crohn's disease. She was admitted as an emergency 2 days ago with severe abdominal pain and profuse, bloody diarrhoea. On admission she was extremely dehydrated and noticeably undernourished. It was noted that she had contusions (bruising) on her upper arms, upper legs and trunk. She explained that she had been falling a lot and bumping into things as she feels so weak and finds just moving around such an effort. Her husband, Dan, is a police inspector and, although he wasn't with Shonagh when she was admitted he has been visiting as regularly as his work allows. He is very concerned about his wife's condition and often seems very angry when talking to you about her. They have a son Tim, who is 11 years old, and a daughter Amy, who is 6. Shonagh's mother and Dan's parents are helping Dan to care for the children in Shonagh's absence.

Shonagh is a staff nurse in the hospital's renal dialysis unit. Both Shonagh and Dan seem extremely concerned about her employment prospects because of her absence from work due to repeated sickness. Apparently, yesterday while the dietitian was assessing Shonagh's nutritional needs she began talking to Shonagh about Tim and Amy. During the conversation Shonagh confided to her that she went on to half pay last month and that the family is starting to feel the effect of this. They moved to a more expensive house so that they could get Tim and Amy into better schools. They had to take out a larger mortgage to do this but they were happy to do it as they both feel that their children's education is so important.

Shonagh is responding very slowly to treatment. She remains very thin and undernourished and is to begin a blood transfusion today because of her anaemia. As her named nurse you have discussed all aspects of Shonagh's care with her. During this period of hospitalisation and the previous one Shonagh's consultant has suggested to her that she seriously consider the possibility of having an ileostomy. Shonagh has met with the Specialist Nurse on a number of occasions but remains adamant that she will not need to have an ileostomy.

Later in the day, while putting up the first unit of packed cells and measuring and recording Shonagh's vital signs after the first 15 minutes, you initiate a conversation with Shonagh. You ask if she has given any more thought to what the surgeon said yesterday. She says that neither she nor Dan feel that she will need to have that done as she is having healing from her minister. She also says that she's really keen to get home again as soon as possible. As she is saying this you notice that her eyes are starting to fill with tears but she doesn't cry or even sniff. She is smiling broadly at you but she has stopped giving you any eye contact.

- Shonagh is giving you mixed messages. How could you clarify how she is feeling?
- Given the information above, what might be the reasons for Shonagh's ambivalence about having an ileostomy?
- What is the most likely cause of her contusions?
- Shonagh has confided information to the dietitian. If you were the dietitian would you make this information available to the rest of the multidisciplinary team without Shonagh's consent?

Risk management

This is a process of identifying the potential dangers facing patients. During the assessment process any possible danger will be identified and evaluated. Following this the nursing interventions will be designed to decrease the hazard to the patient. Common risks that patients face in hospital, and indeed in their own homes, include falls, pressure ulcers, moving and handling injuries and choking. There are a number of risk assessment tools available to assist nurses making evaluations of a patient's potential risks, e.g. the Braden pressure sore risk calculator (Braden and Bergstrom 1989).

However, the process is not only about identifying risk. It's about putting strategies in place that will prevent the identified risk from happening. In the case of pressure ulcer risk this may mean instigating regular skin inspection and considering the need for patient re-positioning, as well as using pressure-relieving equipment and aids. Other nursing interventions that would be pinpointed would be to ensure that the patient has a nourishing diet and sufficient fluid intake. There would also need to be clear explanation to the patient so that negotiation could take place about possible regular repositioning. Strategies such as these will have been identified locally as part of the benchmarking process laid down in *Essence of Care* (Department of Health 2001).

Record keeping and documentation

In their everyday work nurses use a diversity of communication strategies. While verbal communication with other members of the nursing and multidisciplinary team is important, written communication is equally important.

Often, if there is information missing about the patient, their care or their family, the person who knew the information is either not available or has forgotten. Ensuring that there are up-to-date and comprehensive records for the people they are caring for is an essential part of the role of a qualified nurse. Such records can be as diverse as recording measurements made of a patient's vital signs, or a care plan. The Nursing and Midwifery Council's *Guidelines for Records and Record Keeping* (2004) and the *Code of Professional Conduct* (2002) stress that patient records should be 'factual, consistent and accurate' (p. 8). This, therefore, will be an important part of your role as a professional. Indeed, Martin *et al.* (1999) confirmed this: 'Documentation of nursing care is the foremost source of reference and communication between nurses and other healthcare providers.' It is impossible to communicate information verbally to everyone who is involved in the care of a patient. Therefore, an accurate written record means that information can be accessed widely by a variety of health care professionals. Fisher (2001, p. 35) sums this up nicely by saying that 'As well as acting as a vehicle for improving communication and promoting continuity of care, good documentation is the mark of a safe and competent practitioner'.

The Department of Health (2001) suggests that accurate and timely patient records are invaluable both for the evaluation of nursing care for quality assurance purposes and for estimating the cost of nursing care given by registered nurses. Patient records can also be used as a form of evidence in a legal enquiry (Nursing and Midwifery Council 2002). Records of patients' nursing care appear to be increasingly used for research purposes (Hale *et al.* 1997, Ekman and Ehrenberg 2002, Idvall and Ehrenberg 2002).

However, you may be faced with a dilemma when you are in clinical practice, as many qualified nurses, particularly those working in hospitals, don't work directly from care plans. Allen (1998, p. 1228) suggests that this is because nursing handovers contain more relevant and up-to-date information about individual patients 'that could never have been captured in the nursing notes'.

After sharing our experiences in practice with other qualified nurses, we have come to appreciate that much of nursing is an insightful reaction to the moment. As much of the care that we give is often difficult to explain, it is consequently difficult to record. This is both because often we don't have a formal language to describe what we did and because what we did can often appear trivial. It appears trivial because we have been socialised to consider nursing work to be women's work and as such to have little value (Gamarnikow 1978, 1991, Oakley 1984). In our conversations with many nurses and students they describe work such as this as doing 'the little things'. This supports the experiences of Smith (1992, p. 145) in her research study, where she outlines a patient 'describing caring gestures, the little things that make her feel qualitatively different: nurses who recognised she needed to talk, were good listeners, held her hand, took away her fear and had a calming influence on her'.

Such nursing work is very much taken for granted and often appears to be invisible (Lawler 1991, MacLeod 1996).

Over to you

Read Smith, P. (1992) *The Emotional Labour of Nursing: How nurses care* (Basingstoke: Macmillan) and Lawler, J. (1991) *Behind the Screens: Nursing somology and the problem of the body* (Edinburgh: Churchill Livingstone) and write your understandings of their research studies in your portfolio/personal development file. If you don't understand how to do this then you should read one of the other books in this series called *Profiles and Portfolios of Evidence* by Ruth Pearce (2003).

Allen (1998, p. 1226) suggests that nursing records are being used 'as a quality assurance mechanism, which has the effect of indirectly controlling nursing through standard setting'. She also goes on to assert that this produces a tension between the attempts of managers to set benchmarks, guidelines and standards and the attempts of many nurses to provide individualised care.

Reflective activity

The following exercise will help to demonstrate to you the complexity of paper-based patient records.

- List the types of patient records you have contributed to or seen
- Identify a patient you are caring for and write a list of the health care professionals who have been involved in any way with that patient's treatment and/or care
- Where did each health care professional record his/her aspect of the patient's treatment and/or care?
- Did the health care professionals record their care/treatment on separate records?
- Were there any joint records?
- List the advantages and disadvantages of separate and joint patient records.

You will have recognised that all the health care professionals who are caring for the patient need to keep records of their work with patients. However, have you considered that patients themselves also have the right to read their own health care records (under the Access to Health Records Act 1990 (Department of Heath 1990) and the Data Protection Act 1998)? There is also the possibility that the notes you make in a patient's record may be read by a lawyer or a barrister. Therefore it is important to remember that other people who have not been involved in the patient's care at that time will have to gain all their understanding of events from what you and other health care professionals have written in the patient's record. Two very common ways of inhibiting other people's understanding of written patient records are the use of acronyms and jargon. Familiarising yourself with the acronyms and jargon used in the clinical area that you work in will give you a strong sense of belonging. However, you can easily forget that 'outsiders' are unfamiliar with your language. It is therefore important that you always write clearly and succinctly in words that a man or woman in the street would understand.

Key points **Top tips**

- Records should be completed as soon after the event as possible
- They should be legible and succinct
- Involve the patient if you can
- If you are recording something that you have done, said, heard or witnessed, then use the first person
- If you make a mistake put a line through it and date and sign it
- Don't use jargon or acronyms
- Your notes should be objective and non-judgemental
- Always date and sign the records that you write

Conclusion

This is a very long chapter, as we needed to begin to reveal our meaningful assimilation of skills (MASC) model to you. In this chapter we have explored the key concepts that we believe underpin all clinical skill delivery. You should now be able to see that all the concepts to which we have introduced you are extremely important to your clinical practice. We have introduced you to these enablers and examined not only what each of them mean in practice but also suggested how you can develop your skills in each area. There is also a recognition in this chapter that to use the enablers in everyday nursing practice you will have to develop a wide range of knowledge and skills. Some of these skills will be easier to achieve than others; indeed some will need a considerable investment of time and effort on your behalf. This chapter will also have helped you to become more self-aware. You should now be able to clearly state your nursing philosophy as well as your values and beliefs about health and health care. Your attitudes and prejudices should also be clearer to you.

RRRRR**Rapid recap**

Check your progress so far by working through each of the following questions.

1. List the six key concepts that are the foundation for all clinical skills delivery.

2. What term do we use to describe these six key concepts?

3. There are three main ways of collecting assessment data identified in this chapter – what are they?

4. How does the biomedical model of care differ from the psychosocial one?

5. What is the challenge of knowing your attitudes and prejudices?

If you have difficulty with more than one of the questions, read through the section again to refresh your understanding before moving on.

References

Allen, D. (1998) Record keeping and routine nursing practice: the view from the wards. *Journal of Advanced Nursing*, **27**, 1223–1230.

Bandura, A. (1986) *Social Foundations of Thought and Action: A social cognitive theory*. Prentice-Hall, Englewood Cliffs, NJ.

Benner, P. (1984) *From Novice to Expert: Excellence and power in clinical nursing practice*. Addison-Wesley, Menlo Park, CA.

Benner, P. and Wrubel, J. (1989) *The Primacy of Caring*. Addison-Wesley, Menlo Park, CA.

Braden, B. and Bergstrom, N. (1989) Clinical utility of the Braden scale for predicting pressure sore risk. *Decubitus*, **2**, 44–51.

Data Protection Act 1998. Available on line at: www.legislation.hmso.gov.uk/acts

Department of Health (1990) *Access to Health Records*. HMSO, London.

Department of Health (1999) *National Service Framework for Mental Health: Modern standards and service models*. (Executive Summary). The Stationery Office, London.

Department of Health (2001) *Essence of Care: Patient focused benchmarking for health care practitioners*. The Stationery Office, London.

de Tornyay, R. (1971) *Strategies for Teaching Nursing*. John Wiley, New York.

Egan, G. (2002) *The Skilled Helper: A problem-management and opportunity approach to helping*. Brooks/Cole, Pacific Grove, CA.

Ekman, I. and Ehrenberg, A. (2002) Fatigued elderly patients with chronic heart failure: do patient reports and nurse recordings correspond? *International Journal of Nursing Terminologies and Classifications*, **13**, 127–136.

Fisher, M. (2001) Educational input to improve documentation skills. *Nursing Times*, **97**(8), 35–36.

Gamarnikow, E. (1978) Sexual division of labour: the case of nursing. In: Kuhn, A. and Wolpe, A.M. (eds) *Feminism and Materialism: Women and modes of production*. Routledge & Kegan Paul, London.

Gamarnikow, E. (1991) Nurse or woman: gender or professionalism in reformed nursing 1860–1923. In: Holden, P. and Littlewood, J. (eds) *Anthropology and nursing*. Routledge, London.

Hale, C.A., Thomas, L.H., Bond, S. and Todd, C (1997) The nursing record as a research tool to identify nursing interventions. *Journal of Clinical Nursing*, **6**, 207–214.

Idvall, E. and Ehrenberg, A. (2002) Nursing documentation of post-operative pain. *Journal of Clinical Nursing,* **11**, 734–742.

Jasper, M. (2003) *Beginning Reflective Practice.* Nelson Thornes, Cheltenham

Johns, C. (1994) *The Burford Nursing Development Unit Model: Caring in practice.* Blackwell Science, Oxford.

Lave, J. and Wenger, E. (1991) *Situated Learning: Legitimate peripheral participation*. Cambridge University Press, New York.

Lawler, J. (1991) *Behind the Screens: Nursing somology and the problem of the body*. Churchill Livingstone, Edinburgh.

Liaschenko, J. (1998) The shift from the closed to the open body – ramifications for nursing testimony. In: Edwards, S. (ed.) *Philosophical Issues in Nursing.* Macmillan, Basingstoke.

Luker, K. and Kenrick, M. (1992) An explanatory study of the sources of influence on the clinical decisions of community nurses. *Journal of Advanced Nursing,* **17**, 457–466.

MacLeod, M. (1996) *Practising Nursing – Becoming Experienced*. Churchill Livingstone, Edinburgh.

Martin, A., Hinds, C. and Felix, M. (1999) Documentation practices of nurses in long term care. *Journal of Advanced Nursing*, **8**, 345–352.

Maslow, A.H. (1987) *Motivation and Personality*, 3rd edn. Harper & Row, New York.

Maule, A.J. (2001) Studying judgement: some comments and suggestions for future research. *Thinking and Reasoning,* **7**, 91–102.

Meerabeau, L. (1992) Tacit knowledge: an untapped resource or a methodological headache? *Journal of Advanced Nursing*, **17**, 1108–1112.

Meyer, J. and Batehup, L. (1997) Action research in health care practice: nature, present concerns and future possibilities. *Nursing Times Research*, **2**, 3175–3186.

Nursing and Midwifery Council (2002) *Code of Professional Conduct: Standards for conduct, performance and ethics*. Nursing and Midwifery Council, London.

Nursing and Midwifery Council (2004) *Guidelines for Records and Record Keeping.* Nursing and Midwifery Council, London.

Oakley, A. (1984) The importance of being a nurse. *Nursing Times*, **80**(50), 24–27.

Orem, D.E. (1996) *Nursing: Concepts of practice*, 5th edn. Mosby, St Louis, MO.

Pearce, R. (2003) *Profiles and Portfolios of Evidence.* Nelson Thornes, Cheltenham.

Pearson, A. and Vaughan, B.M. (1991) *Nursing Models for Practice*, 2nd edn. Butterworth-Heinemann, Oxford.

Quality Assurance Agency for Higher Education (2001) *Benchmark Statement: Health Care Programmes. Phase 1 Nursing*. QAA for Higher Education, Gloucester.

Quinn, F.M. (1995) *Principles and Practice of Nurse Education*, 3rd edn. Chapman & Hall, London.

Radwin, L. (1996) Knowing the patient: a review of the research concept. *Journal of Advanced Nursing,* **23**, 1142–1146.

Resuscitation Council (UK) (2000) *CPR Guidance for Clinical Practice and Training in Hospitals.* Available on line at: www.resus.org.uk.

Robb, Y.A. (1997) Have nursing models a place in intensive care units? *Intensive and Critical Care Nursing*, **13**, 93–98.

Roper, N., Logan, W. and Tierney, A. (1996) *The Elements of Nursing. A model of nursing based on a model of living*, 4th edn. Churchill Livingstone, Edinburgh.

Royal College of Physicians (2002) *National Clinical Guidelines for Stroke.* Update 2002. Intercollegiate Working Party for Stroke, RCP, London.

Sackett, D.L., Richardson, W.S., Rosenburg, W. and Haynes, R.B. (1997) *Evidence Based Medicine: How to practice and teach evidence based medicine*. Churchill Livingstone, New York.

Schon, D. (1983) *The Reflective Practitioner*. Temple South, London.

Selder, F. (1989) Life transition theory: the resolution of uncertainty. *Nursing and Health Care*, **10**, 432–451.

Smith, P. (1992) *The Emotional Labour of Nursing: How nurses care*. Macmillan, Basingstoke.

Sutcliffe, L. (1994) Philosophy and models in critical care nursing. *Intensive and Critical Care Nursing*, **10**, 212–221.

Walsh, M. (1998) *Models and Critical Pathways in Clinical Nursing*. Baillière Tindall, London.

Watson, J. (1988) *Nursing: Human Science and Human Care: A theory of nursing.* National League for Nursing, New York.

4

Introducing the template and model

Learning outcomes

By the end of this chapter you should be able to:

- Understand how to use the template

- Understand how to apply the Meaningful Assimilation of Skills for Care model

- Think about how you can integrate the components of this model into learning any new skill

- Consider how your learning may be enhanced by using this model

- Identify ways in which to challenge the complexities and diversities of care delivery.

Introduction

The previous chapters have provided you with the context and rationale for a new approach to skills acquisition and understanding. You will have gained an appreciation of the complexities that exist in skill delivery and mastery.

This chapter is the largest in the book. There are two main reasons for this. First, this chapter starts to focus in on our template and how it can be applied to both familiar and unfamiliar skills. In order to make this meaningful for you we have related most of these templates to case studies. Secondly we move on from the template to uncover our model. Like other models you might be familiar with in nursing, it is made up of several parts and is therefore supported with a lot of information and examples to aid your understanding. We provide a range of different situations in which many of you may find yourselves, thus enabling you to think critically about them and 'uncover' the pathway to professional skills delivery and mastery.

It is worth noting that the examples we provide cover a range of fundamental nursing skills and also more contemporary skills that are now increasingly practised by nurses. The examples provide a 'current' evidence base to support the knowledge underpinning practice. However, it should be pointed out that all we are providing is 'key principles for practice' and you must adhere to locally agreed policy, which may differ slightly from the skills content described in this book. 'Current' means just that and you should be aware that evidence changes increasingly fast.

It is your responsibility as an individual professional practitioner to keep up to date. Of course, it would be impossible to expect practitioners to be aware of every single piece of research relating to their practice. However, you will be expected to follow accepted and approved practice in the execution of your role. This makes using the model we have developed all the more important, as it seeks to address the impact of legislation and policy on practice, thus~ enabling nurses to make informed decisions.

How many times are you taught a skill in the classroom only to be shown a 'slightly different technique' by your mentor? How many times do you read a procedure in a textbook, only to discover that it is described differently in the next textbook on the shelf and differently again in a journal? What about Ward B, where something is always done that way because Sister or the consultant likes it? These variations in practice may not necessarily reflect substandard care or out-of-date **ritualistic** practice. There may be a sound rationale for practising in this particular way.

Below we will introduce you to our template for skill delivery. When we teach skills to our students, we apply this template to discrete activities to help students understand the skill being taught.

We will then move on by examining some case studies and applying the Meaningful Assimilation of Skills for Care (MASC) model in its entirety. By using this particular model, you should be able to think holistically about skill delivery. Hopefully, by the end of the chapter you will begin to see how many of the components discussed below are transferable, and to a much wider range of skills.

○━ᴛ *Keywords*

Ritualistic

Refers to an activity that is always performed in the same way, without thought.

The template

We think of a template as a mould or pattern to help us shape something accurately. The template that we use is exactly that. Many student nurses and qualified health care professionals refer to procedure manuals and texts as a 'how to do' guide. This template goes further than that by enabling us to look beyond the procedure and recognise the different components that make up the 'skill'. The template is explained below.

The template consists of the following components:

- What is it?
- Why do it?
- Knowledge underpinning practice
- How to do it
- Reflection on action
- References and further reading.

What is it?

When considering learning a skill, the first most important thing is to have a clear understanding of exactly *what it is you are doing*. Remember also that local policy will dictate *who* can do *what*.

Why do it?

You must also be able to explain why you are performing the skill. For example, it is one thing to be able to administer an intramuscular injection, but you need to know the reasons why the medicine must be administered in this way. Apart from the physiological explanations, consideration should be given to the moral and ethical aspects of any skill.

Knowledge underpinning practice

Before carrying out the skill, you must consider the type of knowledge you need to successfully learn the skill. This is where enquiry-based learning plays a part. Enquiry-based learning is an approach to learning that is widely used now in professional health care programmes. Another approach to learning is termed 'problem-based learning'. Problem-based learning works by presenting the individual with a particular problem. They are then encouraged to find resources that will help them to know. Enquiry-based learning is a concept we prefer, as it captures the student's motivation and continuing need to learn using and developing skills of reflection, clinical reasoning and critical thinking (Glen and Wilkie 2000).

While it is not our intention to explain this approach to learning in any detail, we would recommend that you undertake further reading to enhance your knowledge of this approach. The essence of enquiry-based learning focuses on starting off with something unfamiliar or confusing and then seeking out the information that helps explain or make sense of this situation or thing. It resembles looking for clues to solve a puzzle (Grandis *et al.* 2003).

We have already discussed how, traditionally in nurse education, clinical skills were viewed as psychomotor in nature with little consideration given to wider issues. It may be that, in relation to a particular skill, you need to acquire some knowledge of, for example, anatomy and physiology, infection-control practices and policy, consent and medicine administration. Using enquiry-based learning you can assess the type of knowledge you need to acquire but, for the novice, this should be done in conjunction with educational staff and your mentors in practice.

How to do it?

When you are considering *how to do* the skill, information may be available from a range of sources and can therefore be confusing. Such sources may include textbooks, procedure manuals, local policies, guidelines and protocols. Observing other health care professionals is also a powerful learning tool (social learning). Procedures do vary depending on the clinical environment and client group. It should be emphasised that you must adhere to policies that have been drawn up in your clinical area. You will, however, need to use your clinical judgement to enable you to make decisions about practice that are appropriate for your patient. Of course, clinical judgement is something that you should develop as your experience and knowledge increases and you therefore need to seek advice from more experienced health care professionals until you have reached this level of expertise. This is consistent with nursing knowledge and the concept of 'the expert nurse' (Benner 1984), which we discussed in Chapter 3.

Many experienced nurses have highly developed critical thinking skills that enable them to make decisions in practice. Nurses with less experience may not have acquired such an extensive range of skills but as Cronin and Rawlings-Anderson (2004) point out, they should be able to use a systematic approach to patient care to provide a rationale for their actions.

Although the way in which some skills are carried out differs depending on where you work, the key principles underpinning practice should remain the same. For example, when performing an aseptic dressing technique, forceps may be used in one area while in another practitioners wear sterile gloves. The key principle here is that a 'no touch technique' is observed. Whether to use gloves or forceps will most probably be a locally determined agreement dictated by resources, environment and client group.

Essentially, what is of fundamental importance here is the evidence base underpinning practice. All procedures should be determined by best practice rather than traditional ritualistic practice.

While a proportion of this section will focus on the psychomotor aspects of the skill, it is within this section that you should consider a holistic approach to care: assessment, comfort, communicating and interacting with clients, health and safety, organisational skills and personal/professional development.

Reflection on action

In the previous chapters, we discussed types of knowledge for contemporary nursing practice and briefly mentioned reflection.

Reflection and reflective practice are recognised as crucial to the development of knowledge in nursing and other professional education programmes. Essentially reflective practice means taking our experiences as a starting point for learning (Jasper 2003). Reflection is, however, a sophisticated skill and it is learned over a period of time. If you are participating in a professional health care programme, the chances are that you will have already been introduced to the concept. There are a number of books and journals dedicated to the topic and we would recommend further reading. Many authors have written about reflection and there are now a number of models of reflection in existence. When reflecting on a particular skill, you may or may not wish to apply a model. Models of reflection can provide you with a structure with which to reflect, but do require a level of expertise and experience if they are to be used effectively. Less experienced students may wish to apply the principles of reflection to enhance their learning. The key element here is to value experience, in order to build upon it.

Reflective activity

Think back to the last time you were on placement and you were asked to carry out a skill for the first time. Consider the following things:

- How did you feel after being asked to do it?
- Where did you obtain the information you required to perform it safely?
- How did you feel while carrying out the skill?
- What aspects of the skill did you concentrate on?
- What did you do well?
- What could you have done differently?
- Did you reflect on your performance?

The template in practice

Now let us look at what this all means when we relate it to practice.

We have provided the following case studies to illustrate how the template can be applied in the practice setting. Each case study is typical of situations you may find yourself in during your practice. The case studies represent clients with potentially complex problems to mirror the types of situation you are likely to encounter in practice.

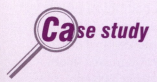

Case study

Mr Hayes's injection

Mr Hayes is an 82-year-old man who requires an intramuscular injection of diclofenac following a fall in which he sustained severe bruising to his pelvis. Eight weeks prior to this he underwent major surgery to his large bowel. Although he was making a good recovery, he has suffered substantial weight loss, which is apparent around his upper legs and buttocks. He is rather nauseated and is in pain. Katie, a second-year student nurse, is asked to administer the injection.

Below is an example of the completed template, which can be applied to the skill of administering an intramuscular injection to anyone. However, as all patients are unique and care is complex, we have printed in italics some of the issues Katie will have to consider in relation to this particular patient – Mr Hayes.

Over to you

Using the information provided in the case study above, what information would you have gleaned about Mr Hayes during your assessment?

Let us now look at learning the skill of administering an intramuscular injection using the template.

Skills development: Intramuscular injection

What is it?

A way of delivering medication to a patient. Intramuscular injection is one of many injections that are given routinely to patients under the classification of parenteral therapy.

In spite of the growing practice of drugs being administered intravenously, subcutaneously and via other methods, the intramuscular route is still used routinely for some client groups and nurses are required to learn the procedure. Student nurses must be supervised during the administration of medicines under current legislation.

Why do it?

- The drug may be destroyed by the gastric enzymes if given orally
- The drug may be required to act quickly
- The condition of the patient may render him/her unable to take the drug orally, e.g. conscious state, fasting for surgery
- The oral dose may not be absorbed
- Larger volumes of the drug may be injected because of the rapid intake into the blood stream through muscle fibres.

Some preparations of diclofenac can be administered either intramuscularly, orally or rectally. In view of Mr Hayes's general health it may well be that he cannot be given the medication rectally because of pelvic discomfort and recent bowel surgery. It may not be appropriate to administer this drug orally as Mr Hayes is already feeling nauseated. It might be appropriate to consider administration of this drug intravenously; however, this would need to be discussed with the prescriber.

Knowledge underpinning practice

- Anatomy and physiology related to the injection sites – dorsogluteal, ventrogluteal, vastus lateralis and rectus femoris – because of the potential for injury to nerves, blood vessels and bony processes

- *It is important to be aware of any local policy in relation to injection sites*
- *As Mr Hayes has bruising to his pelvis, he may find it painful to alter his position, so Katie should choose a site that is easily accessed*
- Trust policy regarding drug administration: re-sheathing needles, sharps disposal, use of gloves and alcohol swabs
- Knowledge of the medicine to be given, including therapeutic use, side-effects, adverse reactions and preferred method of delivery, e.g. Z track
- Knowledge of aseptic technique
- Recording and reporting – *all nurses must learn how to practise good record keeping. In relation to the administration of medicines by student nurses, a counter signature from the supervising qualified nurse is required.*

How to do it?

You will find the information you require to perform the actual skill in a variety of sources, including textbooks, locally agreed procedure manuals and skills information provided by nurse educationalists and practitioners. You should always refer to local policies, including drug policy, which will probably incorporate the principles listed below:

- Check patient identity and prescription
- Obtain patient consent and explain procedure
- Maintain privacy
- Always choose the correct site, needle and syringe (usually the smallest syringe and narrowest bore needle) – *manufacturer's information should be followed*
- Try to avoid air being drawn up into the syringe
- Observe principles of asepsis during the procedure and adhere to local policy regarding skin preparation
- Spread the skin. *We can see from our assessment of Mr Hayes that he is quite emaciated it may well be that to spread the skin would be ineffective. In this situation it may be appropriate to pinch the skin lifting the muscle so as to avoid inadvertently injecting other tissue. Consideration should also be given to the length and gauge of needle*
- Introduce the needle using a dart-like motion at a 90° angle
- Use distraction techniques
- Aspirate for blood
- Leave one-third of the needle shaft exposed
- Deliver the drug at an appropriate rate
- Withdraw the needle rapidly – apply pressure to any bleeding point
- Observe site for bleeding or local reaction
- Reassure patient
- Make sure the patient is comfortable
- Observe the patient for allergy or adverse reaction
- Dispose of sharps and equipment according to policy
- Record administration
- Report any untoward occurrences to the nurse in charge.

Reflection on action: points to consider

- What did I do well?
- How could I improve?
- What background do I need to extend to improve my knowledge underpinning this procedure?
- Is there any research related to this activity?

References

Nicol, M., Bavin, C., Bedford-Turner, S. *et al.* (2004) *Essential Nursing Skills*, 2nd edn. Mosby, London.

Rodger, M.A. and King, L. (2000) Drawing up and administering intramuscular injections: a review of the literature. *Journal of Advanced Nursing*, **31**, 374–582.

Workman, B. (1999) Safe injection techniques. *Nursing Standard*, **13**(39), 47–53.

Although the skills template can be applied to any situation where administration of an intramuscular injection is required, the discussion points in italics highlight aspects of care to which the nurse must give consideration in each case, thus adopting a holistic approach to the individual client.

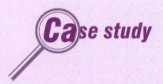

Case study

Mrs Townshend's blood pressure measurement

Mrs Townshend is a 59-year-old woman who has a history of raised blood pressure (hypertension). She attends her local surgery once a month where Kay the practice nurse checks her blood pressure. At the surgery Kay has access to a manual oscillatory sphygmomanometer and also a small electronic device for recording blood pressures. Susan, a first-year student nurse, is on placement with Kay and asks if she can take Mrs Townshend's blood pressure as previous placements have not always provided an opportunity for her to practise the skill. Susan performs the blood pressure measurement using the manual equipment. However, she does not manage to hear any Korotkoff sounds through the stethoscope.

Over to you

What observations should Susan have made during her assessment of Mrs Townshend?

Let us now look at learning the skill of blood pressure measurement using the template.

Skills development: Blood pressure measurement

What is it?

A core nursing skill that provides us with information about the force or pressure that the blood exerts on the walls of the blood vessels in which it is contained.

The systolic blood pressure is produced when the ventricle contracts to force blood into the circulation. The diastolic blood pressure is produced when the heart is said to be resting between beats.

Blood pressure can be measured manually using a sphygmomanometer and stethoscope (described as ausculatory technique), or electronically using, for example, a Dynamap.

Susan has access to both a manual and an electronic device. Our experience suggests that many students believe that using an electronic device is the 'easy option'. This is often linked to their previous experience as health care assistants, where they probably used an electronic device to record blood pressure. However, our observations would suggest that they know how to put the cuff on and press the button (sometimes incorrectly), but more often than not they do not understand the principles of this skill or the significance of the result. Taking blood pressure using a manual device is still common practice in many health care settings and therefore nurses need to know how to do it. As Susan feels she needs more practice taking a blood pressure manually, she could consider using the manual device, repeating the procedure with the electronic device. Of course she should seek the patient's consent before undertaking either procedure.

Why do it?

- **Screening** – to identify and treat presymptomatic hypertension
- **Monitoring** – the regular measurement of blood pressure over a period of time to assess the patient's health status
- **Diagnostic** – detection of hypertension and other conditions in which the blood pressure is raised
- **Precautionary** – when patients are undergoing treatment that may affect their blood pressure.

Knowledge underpinning practice

Check that you know about:

- Normal blood pressure values related to age, gender, race, weight and health status
- Impact of exercise and emotional status on blood pressure
- Anatomy and physiology of the cardiovascular system, in particular how cardiac output, circulating blood pressure, peripheral resistance, elasticity of arterial walls and venous return affect blood pressure; also hormonal and chemical control mechanisms
- The correct interpretation of Korotkoff sounds
- How to record radial and brachial pulses
- Medical device awareness, including care and maintenance of the equipment – *the efficiency of individual models and methods of blood pressure monitoring is often debated in the literature. Remember, machines are only as good as the people who operate them and, if they are not cared for appropriately, they will not work accurately*
- Current research on accurate blood pressure measurement.

How to do it?

Blood pressure may be recorded by either using a manual oscillatory device and stethoscope or using an electronic device.

For both methods:

- Explain the procedure to the patient

- Ensure the patient is resting – either lying or sitting – *be aware of a phenomenon known as 'white coat hypertension'*

- Ensure the patient has not had a meal, smoked or undertaken exercise in the previous 30 minutes.

Oscillatory method

- The patient's arm should be horizontal and supported at the level of the mid-sternum. *Susan could obtain information from the records, from Kay or from Mrs Townshend regarding which arm is normally used. This is because, with some patients, the blood pressure is heard more readily on one particular arm. The position of maximal pulsation of the brachial artery can be felt in the arm just above the antecubital fossa. The arm should be horizontal and supported at the level of the mid-sternum (British Hypertension Society 2004)*

- Tight clothing should be removed and an appropriately sized cuff should be placed above the antecubital fossa and the bladder over the brachial artery

- The manometer should be level with the patient's arm, positioned safely and easily observed at eye level by the user

- Palpate the brachial pulse

- The cuff should be inflated for 3–5 seconds until the brachial pulsation ceases (this is the estimated systolic pressure – do not use a stethoscope)

- Deflate the cuff and place the stethoscope on the antecubital fossa, at the point of maximum brachial pulsation. The stethoscope must not be pressed firmly or come into contact with the cuff, or diastolic pressure may be underestimated

- Inflate the cuff rapidly to 30 mmHg above the estimated systolic pressure

- Deflate the cuff 2–3 mmHg every second noting the point at which clear, repetitive tapping sounds first appear for two consecutive beats – this is the systolic pressure

- The point at which these sounds finally disappear is the diastolic pressure. If these sounds do not disappear, the point of muffling (Korotkoff phase 4) should be used to estimate diastolic pressure. This method is often used in pregnancy

- The blood pressure should be recorded to the nearest 2 mmHg

- Replace clothing and ensure comfort of the patient

- Record and report if necessary the reading.

Electronic measurement:

- Identify the monitor and be familiar with the manufacturer's instructions

- Apply the cuff (no stethoscope is required) directly to the patient's skin

- Ensure the cuff is positioned at the same level as the heart

- Press the start button and wait for the reading to be displayed

- Should frequent readings be required some monitors can be pre-set

- Replace clothing and maintain comfort of the patient
- Record and report result.

Reflection on action: points to consider

- What did I do well?
- How could I improve?
- What further knowledge/information do I need to enhance my practice?
- Is there any research related to this activity?

References

British Hypertension Society (2004) Blood pressure measurement. Recommendations of the British Hypertension Society: procedure. Available on line at: www.abdn.ac.uk/medical/bhs/booklet/proced.htm.

Nichol, M., Bavin, C., Bedford-Turner, S. *et al.* (2004) *Essential Nursing Skills*. Mosby, London.

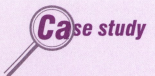

Case study

Valerie's cannulation

Valerie is 19 and has been involved in a motorbike accident. She sustained a fracture to her tibia and fibula. The surgeons applied an external fixator to correct the fracture. This involves securing an external frame through pinholes in her leg and attaching them to the bones, correcting their alignment. However, Valerie has displayed signs of infection around the pin sites and the surgeon is concerned that this may progress to osteomyelitis (inflammation of the bone and marrow). The medical staff prescribe intravenous antibiotics and a cannula is inserted for peripheral venous access. Joe, a newly qualified staff nurse, is on night shift and Valerie calls him over, informing him that she has caught the cannula on the bed sheets and pulled it out. Joe realises that it is crucial that Valerie receives the antibiotics and that the medical staff are tied up in theatre and are likely to be there for some considerable time. Joe makes the decision to re-site the cannula. He has received instruction in performing this skill both during his preregistration programme and later during his preceptorship period. He was deemed competent 2 weeks previously but has only been required to site a cannula once during a day shift, when he called upon a member of the medical staff to check the cannula following insertion.

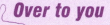

Over to you

What observations should Joe have made about Valerie?

Nurses are increasingly asked to take on more skills in line with the ever-changing needs of our patients and as a result of role development. Obtaining peripheral venous access is a skill now commonly performed by nurses in some areas. Because of its complexity it requires the nurse to have a comprehensive knowledge of a variety of issues.

Let us now look at the skill of performing peripheral cannulation using the template.

Skills development: Peripheral intravenous cannulation

What is it?
Peripheral cannulation is the term given to the procedure in which a small, flexible plastic tube is inserted into a peripheral vein.

This skill was previously the domain of medical staff but is now practised widely by nurses and other health care professionals who have received appropriate training.

Why do it?
Provides access for the administration of drugs, fluids and blood products.

Valerie is at risk of developing osteomyelitis. Infection within bone is particularly difficult to treat once it is established. It is imperative that Valerie receives the prescribed antibiotics. The intravenous route is the most appropriate as it will allow fast absorption of the medication. One of the advantages of nurses being able to perform this skill is that treatment can be prompt and delays avoided.

Knowledge underpinning practice
- Knowledge of professional and legal responsibilities of the nurse in relation to accountability and role expansion. *As a registered nurse, midwife or health visitor, you must maintain your professional knowledge and competence: to practise competently, you must possess the knowledge, skills and abilities required for lawful, safe and effective practice without direct supervision. You must acknowledge the limits of your professional competence and only undertake practice and accept responsibilities for those activities in which you are competent (Nursing and Midwifery Council Code of Professional Conduct 2002, p. 8)*
- Consideration must be given to the rationale for performing the procedure
- Awareness of local/Trust policy in relation to who can perform this skill and the relevant training required. *In order for Joe to insert an intravenous cannula, he must have received training to do so. It must also be a contractual agreement with his employers that he performs this procedure. Joe is aware that delayed or missed medication may contribute to the development of infection but he must also be aware of local policy in relation to nurses administering intravenous drugs. For example, once he has inserted the cannula, is he then able to administer the prescribed drug via the intravenous route? In some organisations, rules are laid down in the form of policies to determine which personnel can administer first- or second-dose intravenous drugs*
- Local policy regarding handling of sharps, use of skin cleansing agents and disposal of equipment
- Anatomy and physiology of the venous system

- Knowledge of aseptic technique
- Documentation/record-keeping skills
- Knowledge of correct technique and identification of potential/actual problems.

How to do it?

- Obtain patient's informed consent in accordance with local policy and Nursing and Midwifery Council Code of Professional Conduct (Nursing and Midwifery Council 2002)
- Prepare equipment and locate environment for performing procedure
- Gloves and apron should be worn
- Explain the procedure to the patient and ensure comfort, privacy and dignity are maintained at all times
- If possible, choose the patient's non-dominant arm for performing the procedure
- Consideration must be given to siting and condition of the vein. *We know that Valerie caught her cannula in the bed sheets; therefore, Joe must consider the most appropriate site to insert the cannula. Consideration must also be given to the environment and patient education*
- Apply towel or pad beneath patient's arm
- Apply a tourniquet approximately 5–10 cm above the proposed site for cannulation
- Ask the patient to clench and unclench the fist to encourage venous filling
- Cleanse skin according to local policy
- Insert the cannula at an angle of 20–30°
- Once the cannula is inserted into the vein, which will be evident once blood starts flowing, remove the 'needle' (trochar) holding the cannula in place
- Swiftly insert the cap to prevent seepage of blood
- Apply sterile dressing to secure cannula in place
- Flush the cannula with 0.9% sodium chloride (Trust policy may vary)
- Dispose of sharps and equipment according to policy
- Document procedure
- Ensure patient comfort and educate re care of cannula.

Reflection on action: points to consider

- What part of the nursing skill did I do well?
- How could I improve?
- What further information/knowledge/experience do I need?
- Is there any research related to this activity that will help to guide and improve my practice?

References and further reading

Lavery, I. (2003) Peripheral intravenous cannulation and patient consent. *Nursing Standard*, **17**(28), 40–42.

Mallet, J. and Dougherty, L. (eds) (2000) *Manual of Clinical Nursing Procedures*, 5th edn. Blackwell Science, Oxford.

Nicol, M., Bavin, C., Bedford-Turner, S. *et al*. (2004) *Essential Nursing Skills*. Mosby, London.

Nursing and Midwifery Council (2002) *Code of Professional Conduct*. Nursing and Midwifery Council, London.

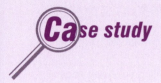

Case study

Anne's venepuncture

Anne Brown is a 52-year-old woman who has a history of anaemia. As part of her treatment to control this condition, she is required to attend her local surgery, where the practice nurse takes a specimen of blood.

Refer to the skills template below to discover what type of information the practice nurse may need in order to perform this skill.

Skills development: Venepuncture

What is it?

A procedure where a vein is punctured using a needle, a vacuum system or butterfly infusion set.

Why do it?

Venepuncture is performed to obtain a specimen of blood for clinical analysis.

Knowledge underpinning practice

- Knowledge of professional and legal responsibilities of the nurse in relation to accountability
- Awareness of local/Trust policy in relation to who can perform this skill and the relevant training required
- Local policy regarding handling of sharps, use of skin cleansing agents and disposal of equipment
- Anatomy and physiology of the venous system
- Knowledge of the principles of infection control with particular reference to blood-borne infection
- Documentation/record-keeping skills
- Knowledge of correct technique and identification of potential/actual problems.

How to do it?

Using needle and syringe technique

- Obtain patient's informed consent in accordance with local policy
- Prepare equipment and locate environment for performing procedure

- Gloves and apron should be worn and good hand-washing technique must be observed
- Explain the procedure to the patient and ensure comfort, privacy and dignity are maintained at all times
- Select a suitable vein in the arm and apply a tourniquet
- Cleanse skin in accordance with local policy. *Current literature suggests that, although controversy exists in relation to skin cleansing prior to performing this procedure, some form of skin cleansing is recommended (Franklin 1999, Jamieson et al 2002, Nicol et al 2004)*
- Ensure patient's arm is straight and well supported. Pull the skin over the vein to anchor it
- Insert the needle into the vein at an angle of 15°, pointing the bevel edge uppermost. Blood will appear once the vein is successfully punctured. Gently pull back the plunger until the barrel is filled with the required amount of blood
- Remove the tourniquet. Cover the puncture site with gauze swab or cotton wool and remove needle
- If the patient is able, ask them to continue applying pressure until the bleeding stops (avoid bending the arm as this may cause a haematoma)
- Apply a dressing if required – *ensure that patient is not allergic to adhesive dressing*
- Ensure patient is comfortable and assist with clothing if necessary
- Transfer blood into sample tube. *Some trusts require that the needle is removed first to prevent damage to blood cells occurring if blood is squirted through the needle. If this is required, adhere to Trust policy and take necessary action to prevent needle stick injury*
- Dispose of sharps in accordance with local policy
- Wash hands
- Label specimen, complete forms as required and organise transfer of specimen to laboratory as soon as possible
- Complete documentation as necessary.

Reflection on action: points to consider
- What part of the nursing skill did I do well?
- How could I improve?
- What further information/knowledge/experience do I need?
- Is there any research related to this activity that will help to guide and improve my practice?

References and further reading
Franklin, L. (1999) Skin cleansing and infection control. *Nursing Standard*, **14**(4), 49–50.

Jamieson, E.M., McCall, J.M. and Whyte, L.A. (2002) *Clinical Nursing Practices*. Churchill Livingstone, Edinburgh.

Nicol, M., Bavin, C., Bedford-Turner, S. *et al*. (2004) *Essential Nursing Skills*. Mosby, London.

These particular case studies have been chosen both to illustrate the holistic nature of care and to highlight discrete professional issues associated with the role of the nurse.

Hopefully, now that you have studied the scenarios above, you should be able to fit together the pieces of the 'jigsaw' and realise that learning a skill is a complex task but it is not insurmountable.

Key points   *Top tips*

- The stages of the skills template are: What is it? Why do it? Knowledge underpinning practice, How to do it, Reflection on practice
- Sources of information that may be useful in enhancing the knowledge underpinning your practice include: patient books and journals, lecture material, clinical placement experiences, discussions with mentors and other qualified staff, discussions with lecturers and peer group and discussions with other health care workers such as dietitians

---

The Meaningful Assimilation of Skills for Care model

Having applied the template to these examples of clinical skills we want to explore some more 'complex' skills, not only to demonstrate the flexibility of the template but also to clearly explain and apply a model we have developed, the MASC model.

In applying the template certain 'key' themes have started to emerge; evidence-based practice, reflection, holism, underpinning practice with theory and tailoring our care delivery to individual patient needs. These themes had been identified earlier in the book as being fundamental to skill delivery and mastery. Within the template we also looked at the underpinning concepts, such as assessment and documentation, that were explored in Chapter 3.

In Chapters 1 and 2 we identified the need to 'contextualise' clinical skills, i.e. to consider the clinical context of the skill delivery, but also the need to consider how you as an individual might acquire the knowledge and skills to deliver care, in other words the cognitive (thinking) skills required, such as prioritising and decision-making skills, and your own learning style.

By now you should be able to identify some distinct elements of skill delivery and mastery that we feel are fundamental – the patient factors, the context of care and your own learning needs. These, then, are some of the essential components that 'come together' in our MASC model. We have tried to demonstrate how some of these factors interlink when using the template. Now we will take this further.

Administration of medicines

The first example of a 'complex' skill we have chosen to explore is administration of medicines. Our reasons for this are threefold:

- It is one of the most common 'clinical' skills that nurses perform
- There is much evidence to suggest that medication errors are on the increase, so we need to make sure our practice is 'safe'
- This skill is itself made up of lots of individual skills, e.g. giving an injection.

We can start to make sense of this skill initially by applying the template.

What is it?

Using the template, the first question we would ask is 'what is it'? The simplest explanation is that it is the way we deliver medicines to the patient and ensure that they are taken correctly, consistent with the patients treatment plan.

The Nursing and Midwifery Council, within their *Guidelines for the Administration of Medicines* (2002, p. 3) state that: 'it is not solely a mechanistic task . . . It requires thought and the exercise of professional judgement.' This definition is consistent with our beliefs of what 'being skilled' implies. However, if we try to make a little more sense of this we can start identifying that it means knowledge of how medicines act, the doses and the routes. It also implies a role in patient education. However, before we start identifying the knowledge and underpinning skills required, we need to give more thought to 'what it is'.

If we consider the clinical context, probably the most common approach to administering medicines is the 'medicines round', delivering medicines to a ward full of patients and involving the use of a medicines trolley. However, there are other strategies, such as patient self-administration, a very different strategy implemented in many different ways, or the 'compromise' where a primary nurse administers medicines to a small group of patients (eight to ten), often still involving the use of a medicines trolley.

If we look at the range of clinical environments, it could be that the majority of patients are self-caring, so that self-administration would be a sound strategy. On the other hand, if most patients were confused it would probably be the least useful strategy, as safety might be compromised. If we were concerned about how a patient might manage their medications at home, self-administration would be a useful way of assessing a patient's knowledge, skills and ability to comply with treatment. However, the reality in busy clinical areas is that the 'medicines round' is seen as the most efficient way of administering medicines, although many authors question the validity of this. This is an example of the way in which beliefs and opinions influence practice, and why we need to be using a contemporary evidence base.

If we were to move to a system of medicines administered by primary nurses we would need to consider the resources available – the numbers of qualified nurses and of medicine trolleys – but also the positive benefits of knowing a small group of patients well and therefore being able to monitor the effectiveness of the treatment and patient information needs.

Often, clinical areas are busy, involved not only with the administration of medicines at identified times but also with the administration of premedications and pain relief, by a variety of routes – such as intravenous therapies and inhaled drugs.

If we add to this the wide range of areas in which patients/clients require medicines – acute areas, patients' own homes (where medicines may be administered by community nurses), residential care/nursing homes – we only add to the complexity of the situation.

Also, medicines are becoming more and more complex, with patients receiving complicated 'cocktails' of drugs. Nurses therefore need to be knowledgeable about how the medication acts, the route by which it is to be administered and its potential to interact with other medicines, even 'over-the-counter' medicines.

Why do it

This is a more straightforward question to consider. If medicines weren't considered important to patient recovery and welfare they wouldn't be prescribed. However, medicines can be cures, symptom relief and a way of improving quality of life, or replacement therapy. When medicines are prescribed for patients it is usually assumed that the administration will be undertaken by a health professional. This is to ensure that the medicine is administered appropriately, based upon the prescription, and also that the effect upon the patient is monitored, problems are identified and the need for **compliance** is reinforced. Otherwise we cannot assume that the patient is receiving a '**therapeutic** dose' – one that is safe and will achieve the desired result without causing too many unwanted effects. The therapeutic dose is based upon how long it takes the medication to produce its effect, how long it stays within the body and what we know about the patient. For example, the patient might be unable to swallow tablets, might not like the idea of taking 'drugs' or might be taking other medications. The patient could be suffering from other illnesses or conditions that mean some medications

Keywords

Compliance
Refers to the extent to which patients follow the health advice they are given.

Therapeutic
In this context, means 'beneficial'.

would be problematic. For example, aspirin is not recommended for children under 12 years old because of its potential side-effects.

There may be many reasons why patients/clients need their medicines administered by carers. They may be acutely ill or confused, or the administration may involve the skills of a health professional, e.g. injection.

How to do it

So far, we have considered the needs of the clinical area and of the patient and patient group; we now need to consider the types of knowledge required, 'how to do it' (often referred to in nursing texts as 'procedure'), and relate this to the individual patient and your own feelings, experience and learning style.

Even if the preferred method of administration does require delivering medicines via a trolley, it needs to involve preparation of the trolley, appropriate timing, the role of the nurse, the experience, knowledge and skills of the nurse, types of medication to be administered, legibility of prescriptions, etc. This covers a comprehensive range of knowledge and skills, which can be daunting to the beginner. Medicines are administered via a variety of routes, and the medicines used in different clinical areas may vary. Some medicines are subject to specific regulations regarding their administration (e.g. controlled drugs) or may be required to be stored in a particular way (e.g. in a drugs fridge). Also, some medicines require specialist knowledge and skills, such as those drugs we use when patients are suffering from cancer (chemotherapy), which can be very toxic, both to the patient and to the health care professional administering them, unless appropriate precautions are taken.

Where do we start to learn this kind of information? You need to start by identifying your own learning needs – what knowledge and skills you already possess and what is an appropriate range of treatments to learn about given the patients you are caring for. What skills and knowledge do you need in order to be competent and what is your preferred method of learning?

As an unqualified nurse you cannot expect to have the same level of knowledge as experienced, qualified staff, but you should be able to identify some medicines that are in common use and learn how they act. However, no matter how experienced you become as a nurse, you will always come across medicines that are unfamiliar to you. One key aspect of your development, therefore, is to know where you can find the information you need. In order to do this successfully you need to identify the 'fundamental' principles that underpin your learning. For example, if you don't know how a medicine exerts its effect (how it works), how can you understand what other effects it might have on the patient, what medications or even food the patient should avoid, or what advice you should be giving?

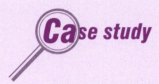

Ms Jerome – implications of medication

Ms Jerome is a 43-year-old who was admitted 5 days ago with an exacerbation of chronic obstructive pulmonary disease. She lives with her three school-age children. Both her parents and her children's paternal grandparents live close by and help support Ms Jerome and her family. She is being discharged from hospital tomorrow.

The evening before her discharge you are listening to her describe how she is going to manage at home. During your conversation you notice that she seems to be finding swallowing difficult. You ask her about this and she admits that for the last 2 days she has been finding it more and more painful to swallow even saliva and that now her mouth feels sore and uncomfortable. She hadn't mentioned it before because she was worried that it would stop her from going home. She says that she is really keen to get home as soon as possible.

She is being discharged on prednisolone 30 mg orally for the next 4 days, along with doxycycline 100 mg daily for a further 2 days.

Over to you

- What is prednisolone and what might it be used for?
- What side effects of prednisolone would you need to inform Ms Jerome about?
- Are there any potential harmful interactions between the two medicines above?
- Given the information above, what might be the reason for Ms Jerome's difficulty in swallowing?
- What will be the most likely infecting organism causing her sore mouth and difficulty in swallowing?

When administering medicines we have responsibilities not only to ourselves and the patients we are caring for but also to our employees and the profession itself. In other words we need to behave in a professional manner.

In considering these responsibilities we are now touching on other elements of our model. We need to add to those previously identified:

- Individual patient needs and principles of holistic care (Patient)

- How you might acquire the underpinning knowledge, use cognitive skills such as reflection, and your own learning style (Personal),
- Clinical context of the skill delivery (Context)
- The underpinning theory and evidence (Evidence) that we have already identified.

We can now add another category:

- The need to be aware of polices and guidelines that should underpin our practice (Professional).

These five fundamental elements support our model. This is just a very brief 'snapshot' – we could identify much more detail in each of these areas, and these elements are therefore explored later.

Our example of administration of medicines can be represented using our model thus.

The 'underpinning elements' we have already as:

- **Context.** What is the clinical speciality? For example, if it is a surgical ward, the main groups of medicines used would be premedications, pain relief and antibiotics, and a variety of charts would be used to prescribe these. In elderly care, medicines may be used to manage conditions such as heart failure, and therefore patients may have complicated treatment regimens.
- **Patient.** Is the patient comfortable with having to take these medicines? Has he/she been told what they are for and been involved in the prescribing decisions? Does the patient understand the need for the treatment?
- **Professional.** Are we aware of the Trust policy for administration of medicines? Do we know how drugs should be stored and ordered, and do we know what to do if the patient refuses to take them? What other medicines is the patient taking?
- **Evidence.** What do we know about the medicines and their potential therapeutic and unwanted effects, dosage intervals and interactions? How would we monitor the effectiveness of the treatment? What observations of the patient do we need to make?
- **Personal.** Learning needs: have we given out this type of medicine before; what policies do we need to read; what can we 'do' to enhance our skills? How would we feel about explaining these treatments to the patient?

These 'underpinning elements' are only part of the model.

- Fundamental to skill delivery are a knowledge of the patient and the clinical area
- The delivery of care should be based upon a contemporary evidence base
- You need to identify sources of knowledge to underpin your skill delivery
- The 'underpinning elements' of the MASC model are: the patient, the context, the student's personal needs, the evidence base and professional issues

We have developed a template related to administration of medicines using a medicines trolley, which can be found in Appendix B at the back of the book.

Using the Meaningful Assimilation of Skills for Care model

You should now be able to see why we noted earlier in this chapter that the Nursing and Midwifery Council (2004) say that the administration of medicines 'is not solely a mechanistic task'. The example of medicine administration mirrors much of what expert nurses do and, like much that is nursing, it's a complex task with much of the complexity hidden from the view of the observer. You can probably now more fully appreciate why many mentors find it difficult to give an immediate answer when asked what they are doing by enquiring students. They need time to be able to bring it to the level of conscious thought. However, this is not an easy process: it needs to be learned and, like much of our learning, it is facilitated by both experience and praise. Helping nurses to articulate these complex issues is one of the reasons that we developed our model. You should also now be able to appreciate that observing mentors in clinical practice doesn't always reveal all that you need to learn. Using our model should help you do that.

As we have said previously, our template is part of the MASC model. Earlier in this chapter we took you through the process of identifying knowledge related to the template to medicine administration but now we are going to take you a stage further and both introduce and apply the MASC model. This will help you to learn and understand the intricacies of an everyday task that takes up a large proportion of nurses' time in many hospital wards. This task is medicine administration using a medicine trolley. This will also help you to visualise the MASC model.

In Chapters 2 and 3 we suggested that learning to become what Benner (1984) calls an 'expert nurse' involves each of us in growth and development. In order to symbolise such growth and development our model uses a tree. A tree has been used by many cultures since ancient times to represent the growth that is knowledge and understanding. We could have used other analogies like building a house. However this doesn't give any impression that it's about how each of us grows and develops, both personally and as a professional. We feel that the analogy of a tree can also be used to represent nursing. When you look at a tree you can't see the elaborate and extensive root system that lies underground, feeding and supporting the tree. Expert nurses are like that when they care for you, as you can't see their expansive and intricate root system, i.e. their knowledge and understanding. There is another reason that we feel the facsimile of a tree is representative of nursing and nurses. Trees are all around us. They are in people's gardens, in parks as well as in fields. Consequently we often either don't notice them or take them for granted. Alongside this, trees don't always seem to be valued by all members of society. Yet they are continually contributing to the sustainability of our world and they return more to the environment than they take out. The same could be said of a nurse and nursing.

In our model the roots of the tree are representative of a variety of underpinning concepts and theories that the expert nurse will have learned, understood and internalised, so these concepts and theories will have altered the expert nurse's thinking and behaviour in some way. These concepts and theories include the works of Carper (1978), Benner (1984) and Smith (1992). The template for skills presented earlier in the chapter becomes the trunk of the tree while the branches and leaves are the distinguishing features needed that are specific to a particular skill in a given clinical situation. Many of these distinguishing features (branches and leaves) may be unique to each clinical situation that you find yourself in. This is because each human being and their experience is unique. However, just as a tree will wither and die without food and water, so will a nurse's clinical skills, so for that reason we have symbolised the fundamental skills that underpin all care as enablers, the nutrients that sustain life. These enabling skills, once developed, will nourish the tree that is your professional practice and help it expand and flourish.

We will now use a specific example of medicine administration to explore our model more fully.

Medicine administration using the Meaningful Assimilation of Skills for Care model

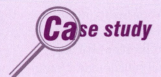

Administering medicines to John

John Seaton is a 25-year-old man with Huntington's disease. He was diagnosed at the age of 22 and the disease has progressed quite rapidly since. He has great difficulty walking and has been using an electric wheelchair when he leaves his home. His mother died from Huntington's disease a year ago, aged 54. His father died in a train crash when John was 11. John has been living at home with his two sisters, an aunt and uncle and their son. He is in the early stages of dementia and as a result he is frequently disorientated in time and place. Sometimes this lasts for around 10–15 minutes but occasionally his disorientation lasts for some hours. These spells are becoming more frequent. John was admitted to the renal surgical ward where you work and you were allocated to him as his primary nurse. He has undergone removal of a staghorn calculus (a kidney stone that fills all the renal pelvis). It is the morning of his third postoperative day and, among other things, you are in the process of ensuring that John's discharge arrangements are in place. They were arranged prior to his admission but you need to assure yourself that he and his family will receive seamless care. You are supervising a student nurse administering the 10 am medicines to your patients. When you get to John and the student begins to check his identity with him you notice that he doesn't know where he is. You check the date and time of day with him but he gives some inappropriate answers. The student gives John his prescribed medicines, which include tetrabenazine 25 mg, and co-codamol 8/500, 2 capsules. He spits out one tablet and one capsule at her. He appears to have swallowed the others.

Over to you

Use a copy of the blank version of our template that you will find in Appendix B and apply it to John's case.

The reflection section in our template would have helped you identify that there could be a number of reasons for John's behaviour. These would include:

- He was having difficulty swallowing all the medicines
- He didn't like the feel of the capsules in his mouth
- He has moral, cultural or religious beliefs that prohibit him from eating animal products
- He doesn't understand why he is being given the medicines
- He no longer wants to take the medicines, as he believes that they are making him worse
- He is using an alternative way of expressing his frustration, anger or disillusionment

- He no longer wants to put up with the side-effects of the medicines
- He is experiencing a period of dementia.

Applying the MASC model to this situation will not only aid you in decision-making it will also help you to improve your ability to think critically. As we said in Chapter 3, the ability to reason is inherent in critical thinking, and reasoning is fundamental to problem-solving. These skills are essential in exercising professional judgement. Using the scenario of John Seaton will also clearly demonstrate to you the knowledge, understanding and skills that you need to master in order to perform expertly in clinical situations such as this. However, we should point out that each clinical situation is different and will need slightly different knowledge, understanding and skill.

We have explored the knowledge and skills that you would need to bring to the care of John Seaton in both text and diagram form so that you can see how to apply the MASC model in this situation. All the elements that an expert nurse would bring to this situation are 'unpacked' for you.

The roots of this particular tree would therefore include:

Patient

- **Philosophy** – What are John's values and beliefs about medicines?
- **Cultural**
  - Does John view the use of the term 'drug' instead of 'medicine' negatively?
  - Does he see his privacy/dignity disappearing as a result of the ward environment?
- **Religion** – Does John have any religious beliefs that would prevent him from taking medicines manufactured from animal products?
- **Ethical** – Does John have any beliefs that would prevent him from taking certain medicines? For example, many vegetarians and vegans would not knowingly take capsules, as most are made from gelatine
- **Health status**
  - Are there any contraindications to the prescribed medicines?
  - Is there anything that would influence the route or form of the medicines prescribed, e.g. dysphagia (difficulty in swallowing)?

- **Educational needs**
  - What does John understand about the reasons for the medicine/s being prescribed?
  - What is John's level of understanding and is it constant?
- **User/carer perspective**
  - How does John feel about what is happening to him?
  - Do John and his family feel well supported?
  - Who are his main carers and how do they feel about John and having to care for him?
  - Is John and/or his main carer an expert in managing his condition?

Personal

- **Qualities**
  - Are you reliable, trustworthy, thorough, patient, honest?
  - Do you manage time well?
  - Have you been able to manage medicine rounds by discouraging interruptions, anticipating possible interruptions and prioritising any interruptions that do occur?
- **Learning style**
  - What is your preferred learning style?
  - Do you have strategies in place to maximise your learning?
- **Social skills – Do you approach patients:**
  - Courteously?
  - Politely?
  - Ensuring privacy and dignity?
- **Cultural awareness**
  - Are you aware of John's abilities rather than his disabilities?
  - Can you maximise his abilities?
- **Philosophical** – What are your values and beliefs about:
  - Nursing?
  - Health?
  - Disability?
  - Patient's role?
  - Debilitating disease?
  - Medicines?
  - The nurse–patient relationship?
  - Holistic care?
  - Patient concordance/adherence/compliance?

Professional

- **Legal**
  - Informed consent
  - Medicines Act 1968, Misuse of Drugs Act 1971 and Misuse of Drugs Regulations 1985, safe storage, legible and legal prescription, availability of keys

- **Ethical**
  - **Covert administration**?
  - Non-discriminatory practice?

- **Human Rights Act 1998**
  - Informed consent?
  - Privacy and dignity?

- **Disability Discrimination Act 1995** – Does the ward environment impact on John's ability to take his medicines?

- **Professional body**
  - Nursing and Midwifery Council (2002) *Code of Professional Conduct*
  - Nursing and Midwifery Council (2004) *Guidelines for the Administration of Medicines*
  - Nursing and Midwifery Council (2004) *Guidelines on Records and Record keeping*
  - Nursing and Midwifery Council (2001) *Guidelines on Covert Medication*

- **National**
  - Are there any National Institute of Clinical Excellence (NICE) prescribing recommendations?
  - How do the medicines management initiative (Audit Commission 2003) and *Improving Medication Safety* (Department of Health 2004) impact on your practice?
  - Is there a National Service Framework?
  - Does the Huntington's Disease Association have any guidelines about medication?

- **Emotional labour**
  - deep acting (Hochschild 1983)
  - Supporting both John and his family, who are having to live with the day-to-day effects of his condition as well as facing the future
  - Is John seen as 'the unpopular patient' (Stockwell 1984) because of the time it takes to care for him and/or because of his behaviour?
  - Positive feelings: compassion, sadness, patience, kindness, respect, thoughtfulness, non-judgemental
  - Negative feelings: frustration, irritation, anger, pity

⊶ Keywords

Covert administration

When a medicine or medicines are hidden in food or drink and are given secretly to the patient.

- **Emotional intelligence**
  - Self-awareness?
  - Self-regulation?
  - Self-motivation? (Freshman and Rubino 2002)

Context

- **Local Trust medicine management policies and procedures** – For example safe storage, who can administer, defining a correct prescription
- **Environment** – Recognise the disabling aspects of the ward environment and make attempts to overcome them?
- **Resources**
  - Is there a student who needs to learn how to administer medicines?
  - As you are using primary nursing, are there enough medicine trolleys?

Evidence

- **Life sciences**
  - Anatomy and physiology of nervous system, musculoskeletal system, respiratory system and renal system
  - Disordered physiology of nervous system, musculoskeletal, respiratory and renal systems
  - Maintaining homeostasis
  - Genetics: inheritance, genetics service
  - Pharmacokinetics and pharmacodynamics: tetrabenazine: may deplete the nerve endings of dopamine; co-codamol: codeine phosphate relaxes smooth muscle and also has a sedative effect on the central nervous system (British National Formulary 2004)
- **Nursing**
  - Care of John following renal surgery
  - Postoperative pain management
  - Care of a patient with muscle spasm
- Psychology – Coping, loss and grief
- Sociology – Family, patient role, concordance/adherence/compliance
- Complementary/alternative therapies, herbal medicines
- National Institute of Clinical Excellence: are there any NICE guidelines?

- British National Formulary (BNF)
- Huntington's Disease Association: have they issued any guidelines or information related to symptom management?

Enablers

Having considered the roots of the tree we now need to explore what we have called the enablers. We have used the term to describe the skills we introduced in Chapter 3, which we believe are fundamental to all nursing practice:

- Assessment
- Communication
- Record-keeping and documentation
- Risk management
- Professional judgement and decision-making, and
- Managing uncertainty.

We have used the term 'enablers' as we feel that this best illustrates what happens when expert practitioners are working in real life. Just as the tree absorbs food and water and uses it in the chemical processes that produce growth, so the expert practitioner uses the enabling skills to nurture the **symbiotic** relationship that exists between theory and practice. As with the roots of the tree, the enablers are used to promote thinking and learning processes and consequently mastery in a particular area results.

The enablers of the tree involving John Seaton would be as follows.

Assessment

Faced with John's scenario, the expert nurse would be looking for clues to explain John's behaviour. The following are avenues to be investigated:

- Exploring with John the possible reasons for his behaviour
- Using an appropriate assessment tool to look for signs of changes in John's cognition, e.g. the Mini-Mental Status Examination (MMSE; Folstein *et al.* 1975)
- John's mood must also be explored using a suitable assessment tool, e.g. Beck's Depression Inventory (Beck and Steen 1987).

Communication

- Using language appropriate to John's level of understanding
- Recognising and interpreting body language, e.g. disgust, distaste, misunderstanding or anxiety about prescribed medication

---

○━🔑 *Keywords*

Symbiotic

When two or more things are not only interdependent but each depends on the other(s) for its survival.

- Actively listening to John and his family
- Possibly needing to advocate for John and/or his family
- Being patient with John
- Being honest with both John and his family
- Interactions with John and his family should at all times be kind, thoughtful and respectful

Risk management

Empathetically explore with John and his family what should happen to his medicine regime if his condition does deteriorate while he is an in-patient. This would be documented in John's notes.

Professional judgement and decision-making

Following your assessment, examine the possible reasons for John's behaviour in the light of your knowledge of John and decide which is the most likely reason for his behaviour. This would include sifting the evidence from John's family, the student who has been working as your associate nurse and other members of staff. Possible decisions would be:

- Consulting the doctor to find an alternative to both the tetrabenazine tablets and the co-codamol capsules that could be given in liquid form
- Setting time aside to spend with John exploring his feelings
- Liaising with the psychiatric services who are supporting John
- Arranging an earlier discharge home for John if this is what he and his carers want.

Record-keeping and documentation

Ensure that John's medicine charts are correctly completed and signed and that the episode of spitting out the tablets is recorded both on John's medicine charts and in his medical and nursing notes. Identify and record the decision about John's care that you reached, resulting from the scenario.

Managing uncertainty

You might feel that you should have all the answers to John's problems and feelings, but you can't possibly have. This is a very complex situation that includes aspects of physical, psychological and social health. John, with the support of his family and the health care professionals, has to identify how he wants his long-term health care managed. If he is unable to do this then his next of kin will have to shoulder the responsibility of making these decisions. John is psychologically very vulnerable and his behaviour may be his response to this. Your role is to facilitate the multidisciplinary team to help him develop his ability to cope with living with his illness. The important thing in this type of interaction is that you should let John and his carers know that, while you don't condone his behaviour, you do understand what might have driven it. It is important that you don't personalise his behaviour, moralise or threaten him with any sanctions. He is not a child. Be willing to listen actively to both John and his carers and make them aware of your empathy with John.

The course of John's Huntington's disease is unpredictable, as are many events and conditions that you will be presented with in practice. This means that nurses need to be proactive in trying to prepare for all eventualities. In this situation, be prepared for a possible rapid deterioration in John's condition. Therefore, before John deteriorates further, arrange a meeting with him, his main carers, his social worker, the nursing and medical staff to explore with him whether he would want to keep having his medicines even though he might no longer be able to give his consent. Ensure that this meeting is documented in John's notes. Discussion should also take place at this meeting, or earlier, about referring John for psychological support.

Distinguishing features of medicine administration in this particular patient scenario

The distinguishing features of administering medicines to John Seaton are the knowledge and skills that are unique to this particular situation. These distinguishing features would inform not only your professional judgement and decision-making but also your approach to and management of this scenario. The distinguishing features are the branches of this particular tree

> ### Over to you
>
> Using the blank tree diagram in Appendix B, enter the information that will complete the enablers and the roots from the information given earlier. Think about what would make up the distinguishing features of administering medicines to John Seaton and use this to complete the branches of the tree.

You may have included all the following information. If you haven't, then you have identified areas for your future development.

- Any other drug forms/routes available and whether any of these would be suitable and/or appropriate; for example, the liquid form might be too thin for John to be able to swallow
- Covert administration
- Concordance/adherence/compliance
- Recognising unwanted effects
- Is patient self-administration possible?
- Interactions with other medicines
- Interactions with food/alcohol
- Reviewing John's medication regime.

> **Over to you**
>
> Compare your completed diagram of the medicine administration tree with the one that you will find on pp. 96–97.

As you can now see from using from the example of applying the MASC model to a particular task, the model provides the means for you to identify the skills, knowledge and understanding that you will need in your everyday practice. As a result it will help you to identify both your strengths and weaknesses and areas for future learning and development. The scenario you have just explored identifies clearly the complexity and messiness of nursing. Many of the areas you will have identified will fit into more than one category but what matters is not which category you fit them into but that you have identified all of the areas. What the MASC model also does is to help you clarify in your mind the knowledge, understanding and skills needed as well as the different approaches and perspectives that you take when delivering patient care. The model also helps to make visible the invisible work of nurses, as it recognises the complexity of practice when the practitioner thinks as an expert does, in a 'joined up' way.

Key points *Top tips*

The Meaningful Assimilation of Skills for Care (MASC) model has four components:

The roots of the tree are Patient, Personal, Professional, Context and Evidence

The trunk of the tree is the template

The branches and leaves of the tree are the distinguishing features

The water and nourishment of the tree are the enablers – Assessment, Communication, Risk management, Managing uncertainty, Professional judgement and decision-making, and Record-keeping and documentation

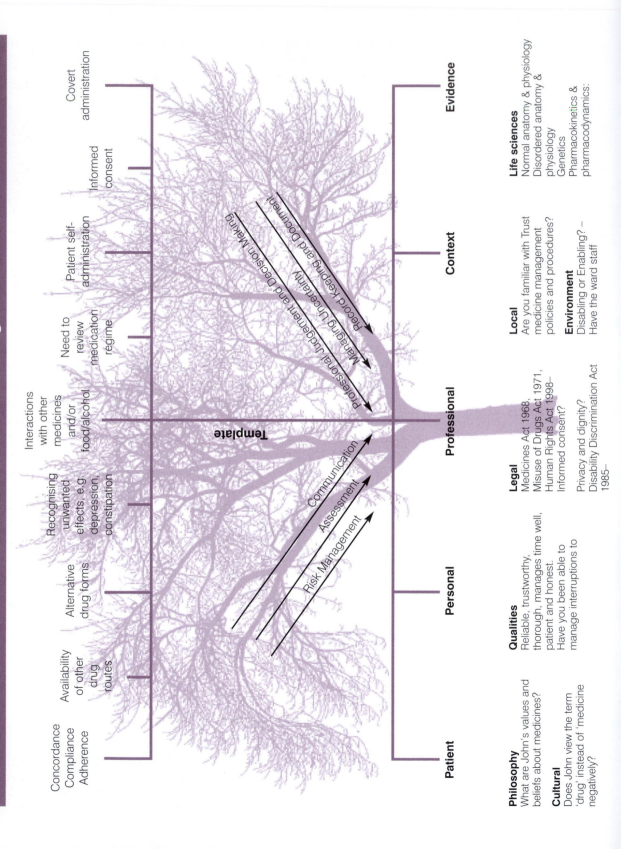

MEDICINE ADMINISTRATION using MASC model

Covert administration

Informed consent

Patient self-administration

Need to review medication regime

Interactions with other medicines and/or food/alcohol

Recognising unwanted effects. e.g. depression, constipation

Alternative drug forms

Availability of other drug routes

Concordance Compliance Adherence

Template

Professional Judgement and Decision Making

Managing Uncertainty

Record Keeping and Document

Communication

Assessment

Risk Management

Evidence

Life sciences
Normal anatomy & physiology
Disordered anatomy & physiology
Genetics
Pharmacokinetics & pharmacodynamics:

Context

Local
Are you familiar with Trust medicine management policies and procedures?

Environment
Disabling or Enabling? – Have the ward staff

Professional

Legal
Medicines Act 1968, Misuse of Drugs Act 1971, Human Rights Act 1998– Informed consent?

Privacy and dignity?
Disability Discrimination Act 1985–

Personal

Qualities
Reliable, trustworthy, thorough, manages time well, patient and honest.
Have you been able to manage interruptions to

Patient

Philosophy
What are John's values and beliefs about medicines?

Cultural
Does John view the term 'drug' instead of 'medicine negatively?

Does he see his privacy and dignity disappearing as a result of the ward environment?

Religion
Does John have any religious beliefs that would prevent him taking medicines manufactured from animal products?

Ethical
Does John have any beliefs that would prevent him from taking certain medicines, e.g. many vegetarians and vegans would not knowingly take capsules made from gelatine.

Health status
Are there any contraindications to the prescribed medicines? Is there anything that would influence the route or form of the medicine?

Educational needs
What does John understand about the reasons for the medicines being prescribed? What is John's level of cognition and is it constant?

User/carer perspective
Is John or any of his main carers an expert in managing his condition?
How does John feel about what is happening to him? Do he and his family feel well supported?
Who are his main carers and how do they feel about John and having to care for him? What do his family understand about the likely path of his illness?

medicine rounds by discouraging interruptions, anticipating possible interruptions and prioritising interruptions?

Learning style
What is your preferred learning style? Have you got strategies in place to maximise your learning?

Social skills
Courtesy? Politeness? Ensuring privacy and dignity?

Cultural awareness
Are you aware of John's abilities rather than his disabilities? Can you maximise his abilities?

Philosophy
What are your values and beliefs about:
• nursing
• health
• disability
• patient's role
• medicines
• terminal disease
• the nurse–patient relationship
• holistic care
• patient concordance/adherence/compliance?

Religious awareness
Do you have any religious beliefs that may impact on your practice?

Does the ward environment impact on John's abilities to take his medication?

Ethical
Covert administration
Non-discriminatory practice

Professional body
NMC Code of Professional Conduct (2002)
NMC Guidelines for the Administration of Medicines (2004)
NMC Guidelines for Record Keeping & Documentation (2002)
NMC Guidelines on Covert Medication (2001)

Emotional labour
Deep-acting (Hochschild 1983 in Smith 1992 – supporting John and his family to live with the day-to-day effects of his condition as well as to face the future.
Is John seen as the 'unpopular patient' (Stockwell 1984) because of the time it takes to care for him and/or his apparent non-concordance/adherence/compliance?
Positive feelings – compassion, sadness, patience?
Negative feelings – frustration, irritation, anger?

Emotional intelligence
• Self-awareness?
• Self-regulation?
• Self-motivation?
(Freshman and Rubino 2002)

recognised the disabling aspects of the ward environment and made attempts to overcome them?

Resources
Is there a student who needs to learn how to administer medicines?
As you are using primary nursing, are there enough medicine trolleys?
Has patient self-administration been implemented?

Co-codamol-codeine phosphate relaxes smooth muscle and has a sedative effect on the central nervous system.
Tetrabenazine – may deplete nerve endings of dopamine (BNF, 2004)

Nursing
Postoperative pain management
Management of muscle spasm

Psychology
Hope, coping, loss and grief

Sociology
Family, patient role, concordance/adherence/compliance

Complementary/alternative therapies/herbal medicines

Huntington's Disease Association – any guidelines or information related to symptom management?

Figure 4.1 Tree diagram of medicine administration for John Seaton.

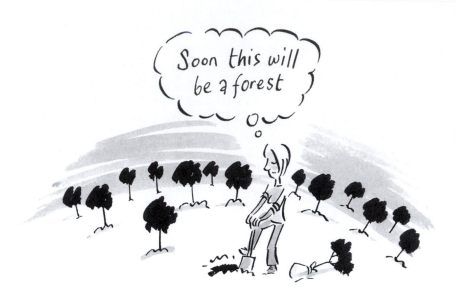

Having explored the administration of medicines using our model, we will now apply the model to an even larger and more 'imprecise' topic. This topic is important not just because of its current high profile in the media and in government reports, but also because it can relate to every aspect of patient care – nutrition.

Overview of nutrition

If you stop to think about nutrition, it's a good example of an area of practice that can be seen as simple or complex, depending on your point of view. If you look at it simplistically you might think that it's just about making sure that patients get something to eat during their hospital stay. However, if you follow the model that we suggest you start to see and understand that nutrition, or rather meeting the nutritional needs of patients, involves a sophisticated group of activities and a variety of different types of knowledge. (For the purposes of the next section we will concentrate on hospital patients, but acknowledge that nutritional care and support is given in a variety of settings, including the patient's own home.)

Food is essential for life; it helps us repair damaged tissues, helps fight infection, gives us energy to carry out the activities of daily living and helps to cheer us up. We can all appreciate the basic biology of nutrition, as we tend to see and hear a lot about it in the media, particularly in relation to promoting health, but it is useful to remember that people who are ill or who have had an accident need different types of nutritional support and usually more calories.

Before discussing clinical nutrition we need to think about food from the perspective of the society we are all a part of. Does our society value food? What has happened to food during the past 30 years? Think about issues related to farming, food processing and production, retail and sales, the media and cookery.

Changes in lifestyle over the past 30 years have meant that food has become a commodity that we were interested in accessing quickly and cheaply. Food production is now multinational and globalised and in the interest of mass production industrialised farming methods are used. The outcome is cheaper food but in hindsight we can now ask at what price, e.g. BSE. The concept of the traditional family has changed. For example more women work outside the home so cooking meals from scratch with fresh produce every day may not be the norm. Many of us rely on meals made wholly or partly with convenience foods, which can be high in salt, sugars and fats. The reliance on convenience foods is also seen as a sign that fewer of us know how to cook. Teachers, politicians and parents express concerns about the lack of activity and high-calorie diets of young people and children and there are increasing levels of obesity within the adult population. The early signs of the related morbidity are evident, e.g. the increase in Type 2 diabetes mellitus. An obesity epidemic is predicted.

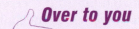

Over to you

List three ways in which obesity can affect health.

There is a growing interest in developing healthier lifestyles, emphasising good nutrition and better quality food. Many hours of TV scheduling are given over to cookery shows, while newspapers and magazines will always include a range of recipes and there's a growing interest in humane and/or organic farming and eating produce in season.

We all have our own personal likes and dislikes in relation to food and different eating patterns. Not all of us have supper at 6.30 pm: some people may prefer tea at 5. Not everyone has three meals a day: some people graze or have snacks. Whatever our decisions and choices may be in relation to food and eating, our family and perhaps our culture, religious or moral beliefs will have influenced them. Food plays a part in our social lives, for example at a wedding reception or having a pizza if you go out to see a film with a group of friends, and family meals. This social and psychological dimension to nutrition can't be ignored. Also, we need to take into account groups of patients who may need care and support as they have a difficult relationship with food and nutrition, e.g. people with eating disorders.

As health care professionals we represent a cross-section of our society. We must reflect on how society, culture, family, etc. contribute to our understanding of food and nutrition and how they influence our practice. Although the population as a whole may be overnourished the opposite – undernourishment – is true for many patients.

If we work in health care we can refer to a long history on the subject of nutrition or, more sadly, the lack of good quality nutrition provided for patients. Many textbooks and journal articles on the subject cite Florence Nightingale and the fact that in 1859, she noted, 'patients often starved in the midst of plenty' (van der Peet 1995). Although nutrition was seen as important, it was acknowledged that food was provided on very tight budgets, even today hospitals are operating on margins of between £1.50 and £4.00 per patient, according to the Audit Commission (2001). Many of us who have experienced food provided by large institutions, e.g. schools, have memories about lumpy custard or gravy, broken vending machines, hot drinks that were cold and cold drinks that were hot, and plastic wrappers that we couldn't tear without resorting to using our teeth. Often a sense of humour was required to cope and we shared this with everyone else experiencing the same problems as ourselves. Complaints about food feature regularly in patient satisfaction surveys. It became a fact of life, people began to expect unappetising food in hospital, many of them asking relatives to bring food into hospital for them and in some cases using take-away meals.

Then key pieces of evidence from Lennard-Jones (1992), McWhirter and Pennington (1994) and the *Hungry in Hospital?* report (Burke 1997) highlighted the issue of malnutrition and undernutrition that patients were experiencing, and the clinical consequences. These pieces of work galvanised clinicians, researchers, managers and politicians into action regarding this issue and dissemination of the work they'd all been doing. A variety of journal articles, learning packages and assessment tools and new policy documents were produced, all adding to the evidence base for practice (e.g. Arrowsmith 1997, Bond 1997 and Perry 1997).

The most important policy document published at this time was the NHS Plan (Department of Health 2000), which provided the roots for many of the practice developments we have seen in this field. It was clear that the public wanted better quality care (Department of Health 2001), meaning hygiene, nutrition, cleanliness, privacy and dignity, and they wanted strong and obvious signs of clinical leadership. These two demands were combined and resulted in the creation of the Modern Matrons, senior nurses who are responsible for ensuring standards of practice and care on wards. With any new role that we find ourselves in we must be clear about our boundaries, i.e. to whom we are responsible and the levels of accountability inherent in the role. In the case of the Modern Matrons, Wright (2003) suggests that they will also require authority if the role is to reach its full potential.

Nurses have always played a key part in the nutritional care of patients. Registered nurses are professionally accountable for ensuring good nutrition and feeding patients (Norman 1997). However, feeding patients (or delegating that activity to another member of staff) is only one link in a long chain and nurses do not have control or authority over all parts of the food chain. Providing nutrition is definitely a multidisciplinary activity.

A large number of health care professionals/staff spend all or part of their day in the assessment, planning, delivery and evaluation of nutrition and nutritional support, e.g. dietitians, ward housekeepers, catering and portering departments, occupational therapists and nursing, medical, laboratory and pharmacy staff. What is clear is that no one group of workers can do this alone; it requires teamwork and good communication. The best way to describe this way of working across large sections of one organisation is a whole-systems approach (Wilkinson and Pedler 1996).

Over to you

In which way does each member of the health care team contribute to patient nutritional care?

Is there any other member of the team that you can add to the list whom we have not mentioned?

With thousands of hours and millions of pounds being spent on nutrition and the true costs of poor nutrition contributing to, but remaining 'hidden' in longer hospital stays or hospital-acquired infection, the government and other interested stakeholders have been working on specific developments to improve care and the clinical outcome for patients, e.g Essence of Care (Department of Health 2001) food and nutrition benchmarks.

Taking some of the themes identified in the overview of nutrition, you now need to start focusing on the impact they have on the patient's experience at ward or departmental level. For example, what might make it difficult for health care workers to deliver care? What skills do they need? How can they improve services? What is the evidence base for practice in relation to clinical nutrition?

> ## Over to you
>
> List the reasons why you think people might not eat while they are in hospital. Compare your answers with those of the British Association for Parenteral and Enteral Nutrition *Summary of Hospital Food as Treatment* (Allison *et al.* 1999), available on line at www.bapen.org.uk/food.htm.

Assessment and planning

The British Association for Parenteral and Enteral Nutrition (BAPEN) identifies several steps in food services that it refers to as the 'food chain'. When developing skills related to nutrition you can reflect on the various parts of this chain for prompts or guidance. The obvious place to start is screening; that tells you if there is an existing problem with eating and drinking or if the patient is at risk of developing a problem. All heath care staff will be familiar with a variety of screening tools, e.g. for falls or tissue viability/pressure area damage. These tools have been developed over time and should have been tested for validity and reliability. One example used for nutritional screening is the Malnutrition Universal Screening Tool (MUST). The Malnutrition Advisory Group, a standing committee of BAPEN, says that its important to make the distinction between screening and assessment and use the following definitions (Elia 2003):

- **Nutritional screening** – 'a rapid, general, often initial evaluation undertaken by nurses, medical or other staff, to detect significant risk of malnutrition and to implement a clear plan of action, such as simple dietary measures or referral for expert advice'
- **Nutritional assessment** – 'is a more detailed, more specific, and more in-depth evaluation of nutritional status by an expert, so that specific dietary plans can be implemented, often for more complicated nutritional problems'.

Although referred to as tools, in 'real life' they are part of a set of forms that you will have to complete with patients. There are

> ## Validity and reliability
>
> Validity and reliability are important characteristics of screening, assessment, audit and research data collection tools.
>
> - **Validity** means that the tool is measuring what it says it's measuring. For example, MUST measures the risk of malnutrition, not personal likes or dislikes related to particular foods.
> - **Reliability** means that the tool will measure the subject/observation/item being studied in the same way every time its used, e.g. 10 nurses could use the MUST screening tool with 10 different patients on 10 different wards. They all ask the same questions and all measure body mass index and rate risk using the same factors.
>
> For more information about validity and reliability read Walsh, M. and Wigens, L. (2003) Reading and judging research. In: *Introduction to Research*. Nelson Thornes, Cheltenham, ch. 5.

specific skills and knowledge required to complete clinical documentation. You have to remember the standards required for record keeping that relate to your profession (e.g. Nursing and Midwifery Council 2004). You need to be confident about the standard of your written communication and numeracy skills, at all times remembering to maintain confidentiality, and combine that with the skills required for assessment, such as listening, observing and physical examination (Hogston 1999).

One particular skill required while screening/assessing a patient involves measurement. To estimate body mass index (BMI) you will require the patient's height and weight. (To calculate BMI use the formula: BMI = Weight in kilos divided by Height in metres squared.) An essential piece of equipment for any ward or department will be a set of scales. However you need to consider whether they have been designed for use in clinical environments, whether they are accurate and if they have been maintained/serviced as per the manufacturer's instructions. Do you have the appropriate equipment to measure the patient's height, or will you have to rely on them telling you how tall they are? Consider how accurate that information might be. For example, an elderly person may be shorter than they think they are. It may have been many years since they had their height measured and they still refer to the height they were as a young adult. You also need to give consideration to patients who cannot stand to have their height recorded and how you would find alternative ways to calculate the appropriateness of their weight to adjust for amputation, etc. This will be important when calculating an accurate BMI.

Once the initial screening is completed, e.g. by a nurse, this may trigger a referral to a dietitian for a more detailed assessment. As you can appreciate, having read Chapter 3, assessment is a complex and sophisticated skill in its own right. The information gathered during the assessment will be combined with the clinical experience/expertise of the staff and the patient's preferences, then recorded in one or several documents, for example a care plan, care pathway, medication prescription sheet, medical notes. This should result in all the members of a multidisciplinary team working to the same plan.

Various supplementary food and drinks, such as Complan or Fortisip, may be prescribed to be used at or between meal times. Some patients will have specific diets prescribed, for example high-protein, low-sodium or low-residue. This may be linked to a prescription for the particular consistency of the food and drink that the patient is offered, for example purée or thickened fluids. The patient may require nutritional support using alternative routes to gain access to their gastrointestinal tract or even to bypass it completely. This will involve the use of one of several alternatives, e.g. nasogastric feeds (NG), percutaneous endoscopic gastrostomy (PEG) feeding or total parenteral nutrition (TPN).

> ### 👉 *Over to you*
>
> To find out more about NG feeding, PEG feeding and TPN, read Gobbi, M. and Torrance, C. (2000) Nutrition. In: Alexander, M.F., Fawcett, J.N. and Runciman, P.J. (eds) *Nursing Practice: Hospital and Home: The adult*, 2nd edn. Churchill Livingstone, Edinburgh, pp. 697–718.

The plan could also include additional referrals to other members of the multidiscipinary team, such as occupational therapists, if the patient required specific equipment such as specialist cutlery and crockery. A speech and language therapist would need to be involved if the patient had difficulty swallowing or speaking. The plan needs to be understood by the patient and all the staff involved in delivering nutritional care, emphasising the need for multidisciplinary teamwork and working in partnership with the patient and their family.

Implementation and evaluation

Once the staff have completed the first two stages of the care process – assessment and planning – the implementation phase needs to be addressed. The appropriate type and amount of food must be ordered, delivered and presented to the patient in a manner that will encourage them to eat. This leads us to the next link in the food chain – distribution and services.

Hospitals, like other large organisations, use advanced orders from menus to assist with stock control as well as customer choice and satisfaction. Therefore, getting menus completed correctly and returned to the catering department on time is essential. Each ward team needs to give some thought to which members of the team will provide assistance to patients when completing menus – staff nurses, housekeepers, health care assistants, student nurses? Distributing, completing and collecting 30 menu cards once a day on a ward can be thought of as an administrative task. However there are several issues that could influence a patient's ability to choose from a menu and make it more than a task (or chore). For instance, their ability to fill in a menu card may be affected by their eyesight, whether they can read, what language they speak, whether they have the dexterity to hold a pen/pencil to indicate their choice and whether they understand the items on it (there could be a dish they are not familiar with). Combine this with cultural, religious and personal beliefs, likes and dislikes, and a patient will need to be given explanations, advice and physical assistance regarding food choices. Various degrees of support may be required the first time the menu is used, or throughout their hospital stay.

Reflective activity

Think about how you react to dishes you've never tried before:

- Think about the last time you chose something new from the menu in your favourite restaurant

How staff communicate options on menus to the patient is important, in terms not just of their verbal communication skills but also of the style of their non-verbal communication. We all have personal experience from shops, restaurants and cinemas of staff rolling their eyes, drumming their fingers on a counter or tapping their pens, suggesting that from their perspective we are taking a little too long to make up our minds. As carers it would be inappropriate to behave in this way. Professional communication skills involve the use of a particular resource – time – as well as other characteristics such as subtlety and diplomacy. Even if you are busy you have to give the appearance that you are not, for the patient's sake. Remember that it is often the patients who have difficulty eating (e.g. those with a stroke or ear nose and throat trauma) who have difficulty speaking and require additional time to express themselves. Helping patients to make choices about food should result in a well-nourished patient, enjoying dishes that they have not been pressurised into choosing. So the 'administrative task' of managing menus involves clinical skills and knowledge and has a link to the patient's wellbeing.

It is essential that you understand the food/catering services provided where you work or in your placement area. For instance, does a hospital or care home prepare all its food on site, or is it prepared elsewhere and reheated/defrosted on the premises? All health care, support and catering staff handling food need to be aware of the health and safety issues involved and the potential to cause infection and food poisoning.

Getting food trolleys to every ward and department in a hospital takes time, planning and coordination by the kitchen staff and the porters. Once the trolley arrives on a ward it can have one of several effects on the ward team, depending on the time of day, the day of the week and the clinical speciality:

- All the staff prioritise the distribution of food and feeding patients – e.g. charge nurse, staff nurse, students, health care assistant

- Most of the staff prioritise the distribution of food and feeding patients – e.g. staff nurse, students, health care assistant

- One or two staff prioritise the distribution of food and feeding patients – e.g. student and health care assistant.

The reaction on the ward can be explained in a variety of ways. There may be a ward culture that classifies meal times as involving low status work for which staff need minimal training and supervision, so it can be delegated to the junior members of the team and/or ancillary staff. An alternative explanation is that, at different times of day, or days of the week, there are not enough staff to involve the whole team in this activity. Meal times and routine medication rounds can occur at the same time each day, so the staff with the appropriate qualifications – registered nurses – will be engaged on medications rounds. So its not just about having enough staff but having the right grades of staff on duty at meal times. Yet another explanation relates to the speed with which a clinical problem can present if certain types of care are not delivered. If problems are serious and occur suddenly, then they must be addressed quickly. Other problems can be equally serious but we only see signs and the patient reporting symptoms gradually. In this case we may cope with the problem in stages – gradually. To illustrate this point you can consider the following scenario.

There are two patients in neighbouring beds in the same bay on a surgical ward. Mr Smith had surgery 48 hours ago, Mr Jones has just returned from theatre. Mr Smith is having supplementary drinks and full-fat dairy products at meal times to increase his calorie intake. Mr Jones is bleeding into a wound drain and has a low blood pressure. The immediate priority would be to check Mr Jones's vital signs, wound dressing and drain – all need to be monitored closely. He could become shocked because of the loss of fluid. He would then require medical attention and a review of the intravenous therapy that he was prescribed. You would be able to see the problem immediately – it's obvious. The time frame that you have to work with is minutes and hours. Mr Smith may have been given skimmed milk in his tea and on his cereal for the past 24 hours, he has only had three of the six supplements he should have because the drinks have not been prescribed at specific times and staff have forgotten to get them out of the refrigerator – they are very busy looking after patients like Mr Jones. The clinical problem with Mr Smith is not as obvious, but will eventually manifest days or even weeks later in terms of delayed wound healing or prolonged infection.

Scenarios like this are not unusual and that is why it is a challenge to deliver high-quality nutritional care in some clinical environments. You need to be able to balance competing clinical needs that have different time frames in terms of complications/outcomes. Prioritising them will require a sound evidence base for your practice, so you have a rationale for your decision-making and the ability to take the context into account – activities, skills and knowledge that can be enhanced by your use of the MASC model.

To reinforce the importance of organisational culture and skill mix and the impact they can have on nutritional care, it's worth noting the following suggestions. First, it is a good idea to have protected meal times (Warner 2004), a dedicated period when routine work is prioritised in such a way that nutrition comes first. An interesting observation made by one of the authors, while visiting students on a clinical placement, was a notice at the nurses station asking staff not to bleep junior doctors during their lunch hour. If junior doctors can have protected meal times, surely patients can too? Second, in relation to medications rounds Mullally (2000) suggests that qualified nurses should see nutrition and hydration as being of equal importance to medication.

When all clinical areas are busy and patients are being moved around the system frequently for investigations, test and treatment, or transferred to different wards to maximise bed occupancy, it can be easy for them to miss scheduled meals and drinks. So, along with an appreciation of general food services you have to understand what can be provided quickly at ward level. Can you provide toast or cereal? What can be accessed from the main kitchens at very short notice – how can you order extra meals or snack boxes?

Once you know what the patients want to eat and how it is going to reach them the next consideration might be where patients eat. If a meal is served to the patient on their bedside table, might they also have sputum pots, paper tissues, a plastic waste disposal bag on the table? The table may have been used, earlier that day, to rest a basin of water on if the patient was washed in bed/at the bedside. So give some thought to the environment. Is it clean? Under what circumstances would you eat lunch in the same place that you bathe/shower?

An alternative space used at meal times may be the day room. You will need to consider issues like cleanliness, ventilation and heating. It might be important to summon help or assistance during the meal, if staff are elsewhere. Getting help is easy enough at the bedside with a call bell, but what happens in day rooms and dining rooms? When you eat at a restaurant or canteen, do you check the cutlery, place mats and the table for signs of smeared, dried food? It is unpleasant to find evidence of the previous meal or occupant of that space, as it implies poor standards of hygiene on the part of the staff running the establishment. Sometimes we will make an attempt to tidy or clean up the area ourselves before we start to eat.

The issue of hygiene is even more important in hospitals because of the vulnerable nature of the client group (e.g. weakened immune systems and/or poor appetites), so you need to do everything you can to make the environment as safe and pleasant as possible. Eating involves all the senses, so you need to take them all into account when providing nutritional care; not just taste and the feel of food but sights, sounds and smells in the surrounding environment (Department of Health 2001).

Reflective activity

Reflect on a taste, consistency, sight, sound or smell that would make it difficult for you to eat or drink something

Sharing a meal with other people can be a pleasant and sociable thing to do. Many patients find meal times entertaining and a highlight of what can sometimes be quite a boring day. Creating an area for communal eating is one way to develop practice. However, at times of ill health, injury or disfigurement the patient may not feel ready for this. They could be concerned about the smell that a colostomy produces, or the slurred speech they have developed after a stroke, or other patients asking them about their amputated leg. They may feel that their confidentiality is being breached in some way. Again, applying your own experience to a clinical situation, think about the time, effort and decision-making processes involved in deciding what you will wear to have coffee or go out to dinner. It will depend on who extended the invitation and who will be at this event with you. We all have messages that we are trying to send, based on our appearance, and we all like to know the social rules of the situation we find ourselves in. The same processes are at work on the hospital ward.

Patients need the choice so that they can cope with the various stages of their illness or recovery. The skill in this situation is to encourage and foster confidence, through goal-setting, emotional and psychological support, so that a patient who initially feels anxious about sharing a table is eventually happy to do so. You will be relying on artistry, ethics and personal knowledge to inform your practice (Carper 1978).

Once the location for the meal is decided, the patient's care plan may require the nurse to give direct assistance with feeding. Being able to feed oneself is a part of every child's development. The independence that we have in relation to the activity seems so natural that we all assume we will always have the ability to do it. As adults we may be fed by other people but it is rare and would involve someone we trusted.

Reflective activity

As an adult, when were you last fed by another adult?
Why were you being fed?
How well did you know the person feeding you?
Did you enjoy the experience?

At our university, student nurses participate in a practical lesson related to nutrition and feeding. Even students with experience of feeding patients as health care assistants have found it enlightening to be fed by one of their peers.

Reflective activity

To fully appreciate what feeding involves, read Child, K. and Higham, S. (2001) Assessing and meeting nutritional needs. In: Baille, L. *Developing Practical Nursing Skills*. Arnold, London, pp. 103–142.

As well as artistry, ethics and personal knowledge you will be required to think about the science of nutrition and the hospitalised patient (Carper 1978). Part of the knowledge underpinning the practice of nutritional care includes an appreciation of food groups, the gastrointestinal tract, digestion and elimination. As noted earlier, the standard advice for healthy diets in adults does not apply to the ill hospital patient. Disease or injury actually causes an increased demand for calories, for example to promote tissue repair. In some instances it is the disease or trauma itself that is contributing the problem and then compounding it.

For example, someone with respiratory disease is so short of breath that they can only eat very small amounts of food. They are too weak to do anything for any length of time but their increased respiratory rate and the decreased efficiency of those breaths can mean altered metabolism and increased calorific demand. So the small amount of food ingested needs to be calorie-rich. For example, mashed potatoes should have butter and cheese added. Following a road traffic accident a patient may have a fractured arm and ankle. They will have difficulty in opening packages and cutting food, combined with having to eat additional amounts of protein and calcium to repair bone, muscle and skin tissue. A patient with Crohn's disease who has required bowel surgery may have been malnourished preoperatively. Altered digestion after bowel surgery combined with their preoperative status can contribute to poor wound healing.

So in practice you take what you know about the science of nutrition and apply that to the individual patient's problems – it's like detective work.

Another comparison that may be useful at this stage is that of the domino effect. Illness can lead to malnutrition, which in turn leads to weakened immunity and the increased risk of complications or additional illness such as infection, pressure area damage and problems with tissue viability and wound healing, lethargy and depression (Whitney *et al.* 2001).

Reflective activity

Access either of the following journal articles to increase your understanding of the risks associated with: malnourishment/undernutrition.

Grieves, R.J. and Finnie, A. (2002) Nutritional care: implementation and recommendations for nursing. *British Journal of Nursing*, **11**, 432–435.

Holmes, S. (2003) Undernutrition in hospitals. *Nursing Standard*, **17**(19), 45–52.

Care plans often involve continuous monitoring of fluid and dietary intake, for instance completing a fluid balance chart and food chart for a specified number of days. It is important that charts are completed correctly and as fully as possible, to provide an appropriate amount of information on which clinical staff can base their decision-making regarding care. The decision to start charting observations or any other clinical activity can be determined by screening and assessment tools, but sometimes the decision is based on clinical experience. However, once the decision is made the chart has to be maintained as accurately as possible for legal, professional and clinical reasons. The importance of correct documentation can be found in guidance from the Nursing and Midwifery Council (2004) and the discussion provided by Fisher (2001). Walsh and Ford (1989) also have an interesting chapter on charting observations, which is worth reading and applying to this area of practice. It is also worth considering that some charts can be maintained and completed by the patients and in a climate/culture of partnership this is an option that can always be included in a care plan.

Finally you will need to think about evaluating the care that has been delivered. Evaluation of a care plan can occur regularly throughout a 24-hour period, for instance at the end of a shift when one nurse hands over responsibility for a patient's care to another nurse. If the patient makes a sudden improvement or deteriorates, a

Key points Top tips

By this stage in the chapter you should be able to:

- List the members of the health care team involved in providing food services and nutritional support to patients
- Identify the key stages in the BAPEN food chain
- Calculate your body mass index (BMI) and decide if it is healthy
- List some of the complications of malnourishment/undernutrition for a hospitalised patient

doctor will re-evaluate medical care as and when required. Sometimes evaluations take the form of satisfaction surveys or clinical audits. In the case of nutrition we now have the *Essence of Care* (Department of Health 2001) benchmarks to use when setting standards and evaluating care.

Applying the model

Putting together all the information that you have gleaned from the overview of nutrition; the more detailed discussion of the 'food chain' and the assessment, planning, implementation and evaluation of care; and the suggested reading material; can you identify and address the issues in the following case study using the MASC model?

This is an unusual situation in that we have provided information on nutrition for you, whereas in clinical practice you would be dealing with a patient. However it provides an opportunity to use previously learned skills and apply them to a new situation; you can identify the key words used, in much the same way as when you are identifying the key areas/issues when undertaking enquiry-based learning or when interpreting an assignment question. In other words, you are beginning to focus and refine your thoughts and ideas. In a clinical situation as experienced nurses you would probably engage in this activity without consciously thinking about it.

We have identified and highlighted the key words we feel are important. You might have identified others. The key words are as follows.

- Hospital patients
- Damaged tissues, fight infection, gives us energy
- Cheer us up
- Media
- Promoting health
- Different types of nutritional support and usually more calories
- Cooking meals
- Convenience foods
- How to cook
- Lack of activity
- Morbidity
- Personal likes and dislikes
- Different eating patterns
- Culture, religious or moral beliefs
- Social and psychological dimension
- Patients who may need care and support
- Plastic wrappers
- Complaints
- Assessment tools
- New policy documents
- NHS Plan (Department of Health 2000)

- Better quality care
- Clinical leadership
- Modern Matrons
- Accountability
- Nurses have always played a key part in the nutritional care of patients
- Ensuring good nutrition and feeding patients
- Delegating that activity
- Multidisciplinary activity
- Assessment, planning, delivery and evaluation
- A 'whole systems approach'
- Longer hospital stays or hospital-acquired infection
- *Essence of Care* (Department of Health 2001) food and nutrition benchmarks
- Evidence base
- Developing skills related to nutrition
- Screening
- Screening tools
- Referral for expert advice
- Assessment
- Specific dietary plans
- Clinical documentation
- Written communication and numeracy skills
- Measurement
- BMI
- Height and weight
- Referral to a dietitian

- NG feeding, PEG feeding or TPN
- Menus
- Likes and dislikes
- Advice
- Physical assistance
- Support
- Handling food
- Health and safety issues
- Competing clinical needs
- Organisational culture
- Hygiene
- Vulnerable nature of client group
- Sociable
- Confidentiality
- Independence
- Appreciation of food groups
- Gastrointestinal tract
- Digestion
- Elimination
- Increased demand for calories
- Malnourished
- Poor wound healing
- Risk of complications
- Additional illness
- Monitoring
- Clinical experience
- Correct documentation
- Satisfaction surveys
- Clinical audits
- Professionally accountable for ensuring good nutrition and feeding patients

In order to make sense of this information we need to 'cluster' it. Using the underpinning 'roots' of the model provides us with a sense of direction to help us do this. The clusters might start to look like this.

Professional

- *Essence of Care* (Department of Health 2001) food and nutrition benchmarks
- Multidisciplinary activity.
- Delegating that activity
- Professionally accountable for ensuring good nutrition and feeding patients
- Modern Matrons
- Clinical leadership
- Better quality care
- Promoting health
- NHS Plan (Department of Health 2000)
- Complaints
- Policy documents
- Nurses have always played a key part in the nutritional care of patients
- Whole systems approach
- Confidentiality
- Correct documentation
- Evaluating
- Clinical audit
- Health and safety

Evidence base

- *Essence of Care* (Department of Health 2001) food and nutrition benchmarks
- Media
- Promoting health
- Morbidity
- BMI
- NG feeding, PEG feeding or TPN
- Health and safety issues
- Malnourished
- Longer hospital stays or hospital-acquired infection
- A 'whole systems approach'
- Better quality care
- NHS Plan (Department of Health 2000)
- Assessment tools
- Social and psychological dimension
- Different eating patterns
- Repair damaged tissues, fight infection, gives us energy
- Different types of nutritional support
- Appreciation of food groups
- Gastrointestinal tract
- Digestion
- Elimination

Patient

- Hospital patients
- Cheer us up
- Cooking meals
- Convenience foods
- How to cook
- Lack of activity
- Patients who may need care and support
- Eating disorders
- Social and psychological dimension
- Different eating patterns
- Personal likes and dislikes
- Specific dietary plans
- Cultural, religious and personal beliefs

- Advice
- Physical assistance
- Independence
- Risk of complications
- Poor wound healing
- Additional illness
- Different types of nutritional support and usually more calories
- Obese/under weight
- Height and weight

Personal

- Developing skills related to nutrition
- Written communication and numeracy skills
- Measurement
- Food handling
- Clinical experience

Context

- Referral for expert advice
- Competing clinical needs
- Organisational culture
- Hygiene
- Health and safety
- Monitoring
- Vulnerable nature of the client group
- Referral to a dietician
- Correct documentation
- Satisfaction surveys
- Clinical audit
- Multidisciplinary team
- Hospital
- Clinical documentation
- Delegating that activity
- Modern Matrons
- Complaints
- Plastic wrappers
- Assessment, planning, delivery and evaluation
- Screening
- Screening tools
- Menus
- *Essence of Care* benchmarks

The value of context specific information

However, nutrition, as you can see, is a vast topic and some of the information can fit into more than one category, depending upon which perspective we are taking. This is often helped by having more 'situational' knowledge – applying it to a context, hospital or community, surgical care, a patient, a group of patients such as the very young or old. If you look at the categories above, there is very little individualised information contained in the categories of Patient (until we start applying it to the scenario below), and Personal, which relates to you, the learner.

This category only you can complete but we have identified some broad areas that would be appropriate for us all. You could take this further. For example, you could identify your understanding of nutrition and its impact on health, your knowledge of cultural/religious differences, how you feel food should be presented, how you would deal with someone who was risking their health by their diet choices or someone who refuses to eat, also how you would acquire this knowledge and develop your skills.

If we now compare this information with that contained in the case study below we can identify further information, continue to identify the gaps in our knowledge, and start to build upon the underpinning 'roots', identify the 'enablers' and start to generate the specific 'branches'.

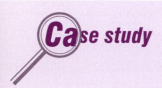

Providing nutrition for Flora

Flora Cameron is a 53-year-old woman admitted to a specialist stroke unit with a diagnosis of left-sided cerebrovascular accident 5 days ago. She is a part-time office manager, married to Robert, who is a long-distance lorry driver and spends most of the week away from home. Flora has two children. Alex and Isobel are both at university, one in London, the other in Glasgow. Since Alex and Isobel have moved away from home, Flora spends less time cooking meals during the week, relying on microwave ready-meals. At weekends Flora and Robert like to spend time with each other so tend to have take-away food or pub meals, but they do cook a large lunch on Sundays. Flora gave up smoking and joined a gym 3 years ago. However in the past 18 months she has gone up one dress size.

The day had started well in the acute care ward. Flora was able to shower, with assistance and then have breakfast at her beside. She had half a carton of yoghurt and some (thickened) orange juice. Flora visited the gym with the physiotherapists Paul and Emma. When she got back to her bed she was very tired but, although she wanted to lie down, she had to stay in the wheelchair because she was being transferred to the rehabilitation ward next door. She has missed the mid-morning drinks on the rehabilitation ward by the time she arrives. Lucy, the health care assistant, gets Flora a cup of tea but this goes cold during the medical ward round, so Flora doesn't finish it. Flora goes for a repeat scan and returns to the ward just as lunch is being distributed. However there isn't a tray for her – as Lucy explains, Flora's meal tray has probably gone to the acute ward. Lucy goes to find an alternative meal for Flora. In the meantime Peter, the student nurse, explains to Flora that there is a dining table in the day room and that from now on Flora will be expected to eat lunch and dinner there. Flora is worried about what she looks and sounds like because she can't talk properly. She is embarrassed that, because she is having a puréed diet, her meals look like baby food. When she gets to the day room she is also worried about the other patients at the table, as some of them can't speak clearly and seem to have far more problems than she does.

Although Flora has started to recover, she has right-sided weakness, difficulty in speaking and cannot see clearly. Alex and Isobel have come back from university and are alternating visits to the hospital with Robert. Flora is experiencing a wide range of emotional responses to what has happened to her.

In order to identify this patient's needs you need to have an understanding of stroke, and how this may affect Flora's ability to eat and swallow. You will need to reassess her dietary requirements, given her potential to require, for example, added calories, and what impact her right-sided weakness, difficulty speaking and seeing and emotional state will have on her ability to choose food, make her preferences known and, in the longer term, to plan, shop and prepare meals. You need to consider Flora's usual levels of exercise and her weight, nutritional knowledge, usual routines and food preferences – for example whether she eats meat.

The enablers would help you refine these first ideas.

Assessment skills

You will need to observe Flora for signs of recent weight gain or loss, measure and record weight and BMI, take a dietary history, establish likes and dislikes and observe mood swings.

Communication

Use communication aids, observe Flora's non-verbal communication, take time, use relatives to supplement information if Flora can't respond to questions, try to convey concern, maintain Flora's privacy and dignity.

Risk management

Assess Flora's swallow reflex and consider referral to a dietitian and speech therapist if necessary.

Professional judgement and decision-making

Use screening and assessment tools to establish need for referral to specialists and 'prescribe' an appropriate diet, food supplements and adapted cutlery and crockery.

Record-keeping and documentation

- Ongoing records of screening and assessment
- Record referral and communication with specialists
- Monitoring of food intake and weight

Managing uncertainty

You may need to involve Flora's family, and specialists, in decisions about her care. Make sure this is recorded.

Flora is emotionally unstable as a result of her stroke. She needs to be involved in care and given time and lots of opportunities to express her needs and fears.

You would have identified and explored some of these issues when completing the 'trunk' or template related to nutrition. This starts the process of identifying nursing strategies, for example the need to address her social and emotional needs, her feelings about eating her meals in the day room and the needs of her concerned family.

And the specific branches:

- Assessment of swallow
- Monitoring of weight gain/loss
- Individualised diet plan
- Adapted utensils
- Food chart
- Need for regular recording of weight
- Small, appetising meals
- Assistance with feeding
- Assessment of Activities of Living prior to discharge
- Presentation of food, e.g. soft/purée
- Involvement of dietitian
- Involvement of relatives to ensure food preferences are respected in hospital
- Assess ability of family to support/prepare and provide meals at home
- Assess dietary history
- Assess activity levels
- Establish activities to replace trips to the gym if necessary
- Organise support at home on discharge
- Appropriate environment that promotes the social aspect of eating but without invading the patient's privacy or causing embarrassment
- Maintaining normal eating habits where possible
- Provision of dietary advice.

These are some of the key interventions that suggest themselves from the case study. You should be able to see how this process has been developmental: knowledge about stroke, refined by assessment of Flora's needs, can 'translate' into specific nursing interventions.

Over to you

Can you identify any other 'roots, enablers or branches' from Flora's case study?

Conclusions

What we have done in this chapter is provide you with a model of clinical skill development that will help you to individualise your care by identifying specific patient needs and clinical environment issues. The model uses existing theories of nursing but applies them in a straightforward way to complex clinical situations. However, like most models you need to start to use it to appreciate its value. Some model outlines for you to photocopy and use are therefore provided in Appendix B.

RRRRR*Rapid recap*

Check your progress so far by working through each of the following questions.

1. What are the component parts of the skills template?
2. What are the roots of the MASC model?
3. What are the enablers in the MASC model?
4. How do the template, roots and enablers in the MASC model relate to each other?

If you have difficulty with more than one of the questions, read through the section again to refresh your understanding before moving on.

References

Allison, S.P. *et al.* (1999) *Hospital Food as Treatment: A report by a working party of the British Association for Parenteral and Enteral Nutrition*. BAPEN, Maidenhead.

Arrowsmith, H. (1997) Malnutrition in hospital: detection and consequences. *British Journal of Nursing*, **6**, 1131–1135.

Audit Commission (2001*) A Spoonful of Sugar: Medicines' management in NHS hospitals*. Audit Commission Publications, Wetherby.

Beck, A. and Steen, R.A. (1987) *Beck Depression Inventory Manual*. Psychological Corporation, San Antonio, CA.

Benner, P. (1984) *From Novice to Expert: Excellence and power in clinical nursing practice*. Addison-Wesley, Menlo Park, CA.

Bond, S. (1997) *Eating Matters. A resource for improving dietary care in hospitals*. Centre for Health Service Research, University of Newcastle, Newcastle upon Tyne.

British National Formulary (2004). Available on line at www.bnf.org.uk/bnf/.

Burke, A. (1997) *Hungry in Hospital?* Association of Community Health Councils of England and Wales, London.

Carper, B. (1978) Fundamental ways of knowing in nursing. *Advances in Nursing Science*, **1**, 13–23.

Cronin, P. and Rawlings-Anderson, K. (2004) *Knowledge for Contemporary Nursing Practice*. Mosby, Edinburgh.

Department of Health (2000) *The NHS Plan: A plan for investment, a plan for reform*. The Stationery Office, London.

Department of Health (2001) *Essence of Care: Patient-focused benchmarking for health care practitioners*. The Stationery Office, London.

Department of Health (2004) *Building a Safer NHS for Patients: Improving medication safety*. The Stationery Office, London.

Disability Discrimination Act 1995. Available on line at: www.legislation.hmso.gov.uk/acts.

Elia, M. (2003) *The MUST report. Nutritional screening of adults: a multidisciplinary responsibility. Executive summary*. Malnutrition Advisory Group, a standing committee of the British Association for Parenteral and Enteral Nutrition. BAPEN. Maidenhead.

Fisher, M. (2001) Educational input to improve documentation skills. *Nursing Times*, **97**(8), 35–36.

Folstein, M.F., Folstein, S.E. and McHugh, P.R. (1975) Mini-mental state: a practical method for grading the cognitive state of patients for the clinician. *Journal of Psychiatric Research*, **12**, 189–198.

Freshman, B. and Rubino, L. (2002) Emotional intelligence: a core competency for health care administrators. *Health Care Manager*, **20**, 1–9.

Glenn, S. and Wilkie, K. (2000) *Problem-based Learning in Nursing: A new model for a new context?* Macmillan, Basingstoke.

Grandis, S., Long, G., Glasper, A. and Jackson, P. (2003*) Foundation Studies for Nursing Using Enquiry-based Learning*. Palgrave Macmillan, Basingstoke.

Hochschild, A.R. (1983) Cited in Smith, P. (1992) *The Emotional Labour of Nursing: How nurses care*. Macmillan, Basingstoke.

Hogston, R. (1999) Managing nursing. In: Hogston, R. and Simpson, P.M. *Foundations of Nursing Practice*. Macmillan, Basingstoke.

Human Rights Act 1998. Available on line at www.legislation.hmso.gov.uk/acts.

Jasper M (2003) *Beginning Reflective Practice*. Nelson Thornes, Cheltenham.

Lennard-Jones, J. (1992) *A Positive Approach to Nutrition as Treatment. Report of a working party on the role of enteral and parenteral feeding in hospital and at home*. Kings Fund, London.

McWhirter, J. and Pennington, C. (1994) Incidence and recognition of malnutrition in hospital. *British Medical Journal*, **308**, 945–948.

Medicines Act 1968. HMSO, London.

Misuse of Drugs Act 1971. HMSO, London.

Misuse of Drugs Regulations 1985 *Statutory Instrument No. 2066*. HMSO, London.

Mullally, S. (2000) The chief nurse's view. *Nursing Times Plus Nutrition*, **96**(8), 1.

Norman, S. (1997) *Registrar's Letter 11/1997 23rd May*. United Kingdom Central Council for Nursing, Midwifery and Health Visiting, London.

Nursing and Midwifery Council (2001) *Covert Administration of Medicine*. Nursing and Midwifery Council, London.

Nursing and Midwifery Council (2002) *Code of Professional Conduct: Standards for Conduct, Performance and Ethics*. Nursing and Midwifery Council, London.

Nursing and Midwifery Council (2004) *Guidelines for the Administration of Medicines*. Nursing and Midwifery Council, London.

Nursing and Midwifery Council (2004) *Guidelines for Records and Record Keeping*. Nursing and Midwifery Council, London.

Perry, L. (1997) Nutrition: a hard nut to crack. An exploration of the knowledge, attitudes and activities of qualified nurses in relation to nutritional nursing care. *Journal of Clinical Nursing*, **6**, 315–324.

Smith, P. (1992) *The Emotional Labour of Nursing: How nurses care.* Macmillan, Basingstoke.

Stockwell, F. (1984) *The Unpopular Patient.* Croom Helm, London.

van der Peet, R. (1995) *The Nightingale Model of Nursing.* Campion Press, Edinburgh.

Walsh, M. and Ford, P. (1989) *Nursing Rituals, Research and Rational Actions.* Heinemann Nursing, Oxford.

Warner, S. (2004) The changing face of hospital food. Speech by Parliamentary Under-Secretary of State in the Lords, 29 April. Available on line at http://www.dh.go.uk/NewsHome/Speeches/Speeches List/SpeechesArticle/fs/en?CO, last accessed 24.5.04.

Wilkinson, D. and Pedler, M. (1996) Whole systems development in public service. *Journal of Management Development,* **15**, 38–53.

Whitney, E.N., Cataldo, C.B., DeBruyne, L.K. and Rolfes, S.R. (2001) *Nutrition for Health and Health Care,* 2nd edn. Wadsworth/Thomson Learning, Belmont, CA.

Wright, M. (2003) Modern Matrons and the Essence of Care. *Proceedings of the Food & Healing Conference,* Tuesday 21 January, Queen Elizabeth II Conference Centre, Westminster.

Further reading

Arrowsmith, H. (1997) Malnutrition in hospital: detection and consequences. *British Journal of Nursing,* **6**, 1131–1135.

Audit Commission (2001) Catering. Acute hospital portfolio. Audit Commission, London.

Child, K. and Higham, S. (2001) Assessing and meeting nutritional needs. In: Baillie, L. (ed.) *Developing Practical Nursing Skills.* Edward Arnold, London.

Handel, C. (1997) A review of the use and benefits of nutritional supplements in the wound healing of orthopaedic patients. *Journal of Orthopaedic Nursing,* **1**, 179–182.

McCormack, P. (1997) Undernutrition in the elderly population living at home in the community: a review of the literature. *Journal of Advanced Nursing,* **26**, 856–863.

Marie, P. and Whittaker, N. (2004) Stroke. In: Whittaker, N. (ed.) *Disorders and Interventions.* Palgrave, Basingstoke, pp. 117–141.

5

Working with the multidisciplinary team

Learning outcomes

By the end of this chapter you should be able to:

- Identify the complementary skills that health care professionals possess
- Recognise the significance of collaborative work
- Gain an appreciation of other people's roles
- Understand the skills required to work in a team
- Identify team culture and its impact on your skills development.

Introduction

If you have worked in a hospital you will have some idea of the number of health care professionals who contribute to patient care. You will also have noticed that nurses are the largest 'group' of health care professionals. It is often nurses who are the coordinators of care, as they communicate with all the other health care professionals.

In order to be able to work effectively with all of these other health care professionals you need to appreciate what specialist skills they can bring to a situation to enhance patient care. To start this process, think about the following:

Over to you

Choose any six words to 'capture' what a nurse 'does'.

You have probably now realised that this is much more difficult than it first seemed. You can identify the skills that nurses perform such as temperature measurement. You might have begun to identify that a nurse listens, touches and explains. You might even have identified that a nurse cares, comforts and supports. If you have read the earlier chapters in the book you will be able to suggest that a nurse assesses, measures, interviews, provides information, educates, monitors, evaluates, documents, interprets and so on.

Over to you

Using the example of any other health care professional that you might have met or heard about, choose any six words to 'capture' what they do.

If you have identified a doctor you probably 'picture' him/her as examining, diagnosing and prescribing; the dietitian asking questions, recording weight and height, recommending diets; the speech therapist listening and demonstrating sounds.

Reflective activity

Now consider what influenced your choice. Most of us carry images or stereotypes of professionals such as these. Is your perception of a nurse different to that of the general public? If so can you identify why your perception might be different?

It might be, for instance, that you want to help patients maintain their independence, because you have explored your own philosophy as part of a seminar in college or university, but the general public expect to have things done for them by nurses. Patients might also want nurses to be supportive, whereas, when you consider the impact of smoking on health, you think a more appropriate strategy would be to challenge patients' health behaviours.

Of course in some situations nurses are also depicted as being young, female and wearing short skirts and black stockings!

On reflection, do you think you might have stereotypes of other health care professionals?

Over to you

To take this further, now consider the nurse and the other health care professional you identified. Are there any skills that, on reflection, are very similar or even the same? What skills do you think all health care professionals possess?

Read the previous paragraphs again and certain themes start to emerge: assessment, measurement, advice, education, support and caring for example. However, these activities could be very different depending on the specialist role. For example, the chiropodist will assess patients' feet and possess a lot of knowledge and skills relating to joint movement and suppleness, and skin and nail condition, but will also need to consider the patient's overall health status.

What we are trying to identify here is that, although these health care professionals all have discrete knowledge and skills they also have complementary skills and that when a group of professionals work together the quality of a patient's care is considerably enhanced.

Keywords

Multidisciplinary
Made up of different
professionals who coordinate
and contribute to patient care.

Collaborative
Of a relationship between two
or more people, working
together to achieve a common
purpose.

The multidisciplinary team

We stated in the introduction to this book that we have written the text primarily for nurses. However, it should be apparent by now that the model can be used and adapted by any health care professional. In health care today, health care professionals are required to work as part of a **multidisciplinary** team, which brings cross-discipline expertise to patients in a coordinated and **collaborative** way. The concept of working in a multidisciplinary team in health care is not new, but in contemporary health care it has become a major focus. In this chapter we will explore some of the reasons for this. We hope to uncover some of the theoretical, philosophical and practical components underpinning collaborative work. We will offer our model as a framework to enable you to explore an activity that involves the skill and expertise of the collaborative health care team: discharge planning.

So what do we mean by the term 'multidisciplinary' and why do we need collaborative work? Historically, health care was delivered by individuals with discrete professional roles. However, health care professionals realised that a more integrated approach was required to address the physiological, psychological, sociological and spiritual needs of patients. Putting the patient at the centre of care was paramount, taking into account partnerships with carers too. Pivotal to this were developments in policy, practice and education (Glen and Leiba 2002). The NHS Plan (Department of Health 2000a) mapped out a strategy to address the health care needs of the population by proposing, among other things, new roles for nurses, generic health care workers and roles that push back the boundaries and discrete identities of health care workers. This will obviously impact on the way in which these individuals are educated. At present there is a drive for interprofessional education and you may have already been exposed to this on your particular programme. Often, students from different professional groups undertake shared learning in an effort to promote teamwork and a shared understanding of each other's roles.

However before we go any further in terms of discussing roles and multidisciplinary work, it's important to understand what a team is and the impact it can have on clinical practice and care.

What's a team?

A team is a group of people who work together to achieve specific goals. How the individuals in the group interact will determine how effective the team is as a whole. Borill *et al.* (2001) cite a more detailed definition of the word team, based on the work of Mohram *et al.* (1995). Looking at this definition, it's worth considering some of the key expressions, such as 'mutually accountable', 'share goals', 'affects the results', 'responsibility for each other'. To apply these terms to a clinical scenario we can use the example of mobilising patients after surgery for a hip replacement. The surgeon will need to inform the physiotherapists and nursing staff about any special characteristics of the patient's postoperative programme and prescribe a postoperative regime. The physiotherapists will need to teach the patient specific postoperative exercises and how to move in bed, transfer to a chair, use crutches and negotiate stairs. Experienced orthopaedic nurses will also know how to teach these techniques and, in the absence of the physiotherapists, will reinforce the advice and exercises taught. The nurses will manage the patient's pain in conjunction with the anaesthetist. Good pain control will encourage the patient to mobilise quickly.

All these professionals need to have the same goal – a mobile patient, with a stable prosthetic hip, who knows what to do to maintain the stability of the new joint. Although the consultant will be ultimately accountable for the patient's care, all the registered professionals involved are personally accountable for their own practice, as stipulated by their own professional body.

It only takes one member of this team not to communicate clearly or to omit an aspect of care and the chances of a positive clinical outcome could be reduced. For instance, the medical staff forget to prescribe anticoagulants (used to reduce the chance of the patient developing a deep vein thrombosis – DVT). This is a genuine oversight. Alternatively, the nursing staff do not use all the prescriptions for pain medication. They are avoiding opiates because they are scared that the patient will experience respiratory depression, even though his respiratory rate is 14 breaths a minute and his oxygen saturation is 98%. As his pain is not controlled, the patient finds remobilising difficult. This demonstrates a poor evidence base for practice.

The physiotherapists didn't get the opportunity to teach the patient deep breathing exercises preoperatively. Every time they came to the ward the patient was either in the X-ray department, having an electrocardiogram (ECG) or having a meal. This is related to the way services are structured and designed. Had the patient attended an pre-admission assessment clinic then all these investigations would have been complete before his arrival on the ward. This would have provided more time for him to work with the physiotherapists. With delays in treatment and health promotion this patient could end up with a chest infection or a DVT.

We have noted all the following phenomena: risk management, evidence, context, decision-making, as being important to the way this team is working. All these are part of the MASC model.

Teams need to manage risk together (Department of Health 2000b). For instance, the nurses could have spotted that the prescription for the anticoagulant was missing and told the doctor. The anaesthetist could prompt the nurses to administer more opiates and support the nurses in doing this with some additional information about the statistical chances of respiratory depression and the parameters for the patient's vital signs that would show that a problem was starting to develop. The nurses might be able to reschedule the patient's ECG so that the physiotherapists could carry out their preoperative assessment and teaching. Being a good team player means that all the staff have to be aware of each other's roles and know all the steps in the patient's care pathway.

The team required to remobilise postoperative patients will be a permanent one. Even though the staff are based in different departments they will work together regularly on a specific ward. Regardless of who fills a specific post or role, the numbers and types of role will remain stable. Other teams are temporary. Project management is used to implement specific changes in clinical areas, for instance designing a new department or deciding what computer software to buy for a clinical records department. The team will draw on a range of staff, experts and managers, for a specified period. There are also different degrees of formality ascribed to teams. A pain management team will have a specific remit, budget and staffing requirements; it will also have a set of clinical outcomes to achieve. A journal club set up by several staff from neighbouring wards will provide information and peer support. It has a transient membership and no formal remit from the Trust. Although the members of this club don't see themselves as a team, other staff do.

As well as giving some consideration to the levels of formality and permanency of a team, you may also be experiencing a 'layering' effect in terms of team membership. Working in health care organisations means that you'll belong to more than one team at any time. For instance one registered nurse could be a member of all of the following teams:

- Team nurse, North Team – formal, permanent
- Staff nurse, Primrose Ward – formal, permanent
- Staff nurse, nutrition link nurse – formal, permanent

- Orthopaedic Department entry, karaoke competition – informal, temporary
- Postgraduate research interest group – informal, indeterminate
- Clinical effectiveness secondment – formal, temporary.

The layering effect is going to call for serious analysis on your part. What skills will you require for each specific team? Conflict management, emotional intelligence, risk management and decision-making are just a few examples of team skills. There will be a personal, professional and contextual dimension to the team's remit and your contribution. Essentially, all the key components of the MASC model can be used to map the skills you currently possess as a team player (and those that you need to develop).

> ## Over to you
>
> List all the teams you belong to.
> What role do you play?
> How formal is the team?
> How permanent is your membership?

Team culture

Keywords

Culture

The customs, traditions, rituals and values shared by a particular group, which will influence their beliefs, behaviour and function.

An important part of your analysis of teamwork is the concept of team '**culture**'. Not only do you require skills to work in a team, but a team culture could either encourage or stifle your skills development. To help you start thinking about culture we have used a metaphor suggested by the NHS Modernisation Agency (2004, p. 8): If your team were a car, what car would it be and why?

The car

It has 140 000 miles on the clock. Although it has five doors, no two are the same colour. Every panel is rusty and the rust is visible from the other side of the street. This car starts if and when it wants to and doesn't start at all in damp or wet conditions. It has very poor fuel economy. The brake hoses are nearly corroded, so it's dangerous for its driver, passengers and other road users.

The team

This team has worked together for a very long time. They are complacent about their skills; everyone knows their job 'inside out'. Although there are five staff they look and behave like individuals, even though their roles are complementary. Their evidence base has started to decay – no one in the team has attended any form of training or an educational update in 7 months. They are not following Trust procedures and are making their own decisions about how they will work and deliver care. This team will eventually harm a patient colleague or one of its own members, if changes are not made.

It is unlikely that you would want to work with this team and it is even more unlikely that you would learn anything positive by doing so. We can learn from negative experiences but that requires appropriate levels of support and the opportunity to debrief and reflect. This team's culture could result in a student observing poor practice, working without appropriate supervision and having no links made between professional values and behaviour.

Of course there are many clinical teams where the cultures are positive, nurturing and safe for patients and students alike. It is worth remembering the theories advocated by Bandura (1977) and Vygotsky (1978) described in Chapter 2. They discussed social and situated learning respectively, involving role modelling and learning by interacting with others in a work environment. This links to the concept of team culture in as much as team culture will determine many of the characteristics of the environment and situations learners find themselves in. Team culture can influence your skills and practice development (Walsh and Walsh 1998).

Reflective activity

What types of team culture will make it easy for you to develop skills (NHS Modernisation Agency 2004)?

Reflective activity

Think about a placement where you have worked recently. This could be in the hospital setting or in the community. Make a list of the individuals who made up the multidisciplinary team.

How the multidisciplinary team operates

Because you are preparing to enter the arena of the multidisciplinary team, you must recognise the significance and relevance of participating in such a group. You must also develop an appreciation of the role of the nurse and the role of others involved in the team both in terms of professional responsibility (Nursing and Midwifery Council 2002) and social function.

This is a complex process because, historically, allied health professions, and in particular nurses, have been viewed as subservient to medicine. In the past, decisions were made predominantly by those with historical/authority-based power – doctors and managers (Daly *et al.* 2002). The definitive explanation of what constitutes a profession compounds this and, furthermore, nurses in particular have always had difficulty in articulating what they do. Tradition also impacts on the function of a multidisciplinary team in terms of expected roles and their function. For example, historically, the nurse was often perceived as the doctor's 'handmaiden'. You will discover throughout your education and experience that there are often assumptions made about established roles and hierarchy. None the less, in health care today, nurses and the allied health professions are developing roles that require them to take on increased responsibility and, as a consequence, they are much more proactive in the decision-making process.

Over to you

Think about the advantages and potential disadvantages of working in a multidisciplinary team. You might want to perform a SWOB analysis:

- Strengths
- Weaknesses
- Opportunities
- Barriers.

So now we have established what a multidisciplinary team is. Let us now discuss some of the factors associated with effective teamwork.

Communication

We discussed the concept of communication in Chapter 3. You will realise that communication is an essential enabling skill for all health care professionals. However, communication is an umbrella term for a skill that is multifaceted. Communication is an essential element in teamwork in order to ensure that everyone shares a sense of common purpose. Good communication is a prerequisite for a patient's well coordinated journey from admission to discharge. This should extend not only between individuals but also between agencies and organisations involved in patient care.

Communication is considered in much of the literature prepared for health care professionals. Written as well as verbal communication is an integral part of collaborative work. In some clinical areas, multidisciplinary documentation is used, for example integrated care pathways, care maps and multidisciplinary care plans. These are terms given to documentation that is used by a variety of professionals involved in care of the patient in an effort to facilitate seamless care. What is important for you to remember is that, when you are working as part of a multidisciplinary team, your contribution is important and crucial to the care process. In order to articulate this you must have well-developed communication skills. It is useful to remember that the person who is the loudest is not necessarily the best communicator. On the other hand, the quiet person should not be viewed as a poor communicator and the art of listening is a powerful licence to enable effective communication.

Role identity

Each individual in an effective team will have an expected role that is understood by others in the group, although the level of understanding may be quite superficial or assumed. The effectiveness of a team can be compromised when a team member assumes a role that is different from their perceived role. Historically, leading healthcare teams has always been the domain of medical staff, and this is well documented in the literature (Howkins and Thornton 2002, Daly et al 2002, Walsh 2001) However, today the shift in health care is from professional autonomy to 'user' need and the context in which teams function may influence who takes the lead. For example, the balance of leadership may be significantly different in each of the following environments: nurse-led clinics, midwifery-led units, rehabilitation units, primary care setting, secondary care setting.

It can be argued that, at any particular time, people never truly manifest the whole of their identity (Hornby and Atkins 2000). As individuals, we all have our own personal roles – mother, wife, husband, child, even patient/service user. In our professional roles we may not become conscious of our personal role unless circumstance draws us either consciously or subconsciously to the latter. What is important for effective collaborative working is that each individual is recognised for the positive contribution that their role brings to the caring process, whether consultant surgeon, radiographer, physiotherapist, nurse or dietitian. Of course, within a team, regardless of professional role, individuals do not all possess the same skills. Belbin, in his seminal work (1993), developed ideas about the functions individuals have in teams.

Belbin linked an individual's personality traits with group role behaviour and related both to their performance in a team. He suggested that we have a functional role and a team role; sometimes they are compatible and sometimes they are not. Your functional role might be that of head of the physiotherapy department and your team role might be that of coordinator. Belbin (1993, p. 23) described the coordinator as someone who 'clarifies goals, promotes decision-making, delegates well'. The resulting compatibility should mean that you enjoy your job and are a productive head of department. There are eight more team roles, each with a set of strengths and allowable weaknesses. Even without access to the correct assessment tools, some of the characteristics of certain roles might seem as if they'd apply to you.

Take the example of two senior staff nurses working in the Theatre Department of a district general hospital. Both have the same functional role but are quite different in terms of their team role.

Dave is an extrovert and really chatty. He always gets the theatre porters to collect patients without ever having to wait more than 3 minutes. If he is **circulating** during an operating list he always knows where to find extra sterile supplies and is always able to coax the Supplies Department to send extra pillows to the Recovery Room. He does tend to wander off when it's quiet, particularly if he has had to do the same thing too often on consecutive shifts, for instance four 8-hour shifts in Recovery. He calls this 'doing his rounds', or 'I'm just returning equipment'. It means he's going to have a chat with the staff on the High-Dependency Unit (HDU), or Accident & Emergency (A&E), or to the Supplies Department to say thank you. By the time he gets back to theatre he'll be able to tell the rest of the team that there are two beds on HDU, the A&E staff are dealing with admissions from a road traffic accident and it looks like there will be emergency orthopaedic cases requiring surgery. The sterile supplies department are rushed off their feet, so it's not worth asking about sterilising the extra instrument trays for another couple of hours. Meanwhile, Stella, the department manager, has been looking for Dave, as he's been out of the department for 45 minutes.

Keywords

Circulate

A term used to describe the role performed by a nurse or ODA/ODP. It involves maintaining a sterile operating field, supplying equipment to the staff performing the operation, counting smaller items of equipment such as sutures/needles and swabs and assisting in calculating fluid loss.

Jacqui is a quiet, helpful and very professional staff nurse. One of her strengths is that she has very good listening skills. Whenever anyone in the department has a problem, either at home or at work, they know that they can always talk about it to Jacqui and that she will maintain their confidentiality. Stella always allocates Jacqui to manage Theatre 1 on Monday mornings. That is where Mr Smith deals with his general surgical list. If the start time of the list is delayed for any reason, Mr Smith becomes impatient, occasionally barking orders at the nursing staff and operating department assistants/practitioners (ODA/ODPs). This has upset some of the team in the past. Jacqui can always keep the list running to time and makes sure that everyone gets a coffee break. She keeps everyone happy and calm. Within the department she is thought to have the best skills for managing routine lists, but she's hopeless at managing emergency cases. As Jacqui is a senior staff nurse she often deputises for Stella. Although Jacqui tends to be very professional, Stella has noticed that Sue, Barbara and Diane (the E grades) are always able to make Jacqui redraft the duty roster when Stella is not around.

Over to you

Find and read Meredith Belbin's *Team Roles at Work* (1993). Can you identify:

- Dave's team role and skills
- Jacqui's team role and skills?

Discharge planning

We have chosen discharge planning as the focus of skill development in this chapter as it is an important aspect of care that requires the expertise of a number of health care professionals. This is the part of the book where you may consider learning a particular skill in the company of others, taking into account their philosophy, expertise and role identity. It might be helpful to relate this exercise to a particular patient whose discharge planning you have been involved with.

Discharge planning is a major issue in health care. For a number of years now, probably as a result of an increase in day surgery and the increasing demands on beds, patients are discharged from hospital almost immediately after treatment. It is therefore imperative that health care professionals achieve effective and timely discharge for patients.

You can refer to our 'blank' tree diagram to help you think about the issues involved in planning the discharge of a patient (see Appendix B). We have provided the headings but now it's over to you to complete them. Think about each concept and consider the responsibilities in relation to your own particular role. We have provide some clues to help you piece together the whole picture. Check your tree with our information below:

Roots

Patient

- Consider the cultural and social background to which your patient belongs.
- What personal characteristics does your patient present with? For example, are they independent, are they confident, do they like to be in control of their lives or do they rely heavily on others, are they compliant?
- What kind of expectations does your patient have about their discharge?
- What are their educational needs in relation to their health and are they able to retain information?
- Does the patient have any religious beliefs that may influence care, for example Jehovah's Witness, Jewish, Muslim?

Personal

- Consider your own individual learning style: do you prefer learning independently or with others?
- What are your own beliefs about illness, death and bereavement?
- How well do you work with other members of a team?
- How would you describe yourself to others in terms of being a 'team player'?
- Have you any preconceived ideas about roles and responsibilities?
- How do you get along with other people?
- How confident are you at putting forward your own ideas or challenging those of others?

Professional

- In terms of legal and professional issues, what are your responsibilities in terms of ensuring a safe and effective discharge?

- What local and national policies govern discharge planning?
- Who is ultimately responsible for the discharge of a patient?
- Are there any ethical issues apparent in relation to discharge of patients: for example, consider here pressure on beds, waiting lists, staff shortages?
- What might the consequences be of a poorly planned discharge?

Context

- Think about resources and services required.
- What sort of organisations or agencies may be required to ensure effective discharge planning of your patient?
- Do you need to consider involving carers/family members and, if so, what are their needs?
- Is the patient being discharged to their own home or local authority care?
- What is the relationship at the primary/secondary care interface?

Evidence

- What do you already know about discharge planning?
- What sources of information will you require to enhance your existing knowledge and where can this be obtained?
- What does the Department of Health say about discharge planning?
- What do you understand about the patient's disease/disorder and the associated trajectory?

Enablers

Assessment

We have discussed the importance of the assessment process during the patient experience and this also applies to the discharge planning process. You may need to give consideration to particular assessment tools such as pain, tissue viability, risk of falls, deep vein thrombosis and nutrition. If your patient has undergone a surgical procedure, you must ensure that they are fully recovered from the anaesthetic before contemplating discharge.

Communication

Communication is essential for a smooth and efficient discharge. It is vital that agencies, organisations and individuals communicate with one another. This should commence during the admission process and continue through referral to actual discharge. It is also essential that you communicate with the patient and their carer(s). Communication can be verbal but written documentation will also be required. Your patient may need information about follow-up appointments, treatment, medicines and contact numbers, as well as instruction about the use of any aids or prosthetics.

The way in which you speak to patients is very important. You must avoid using terminology that patients will not understand. You must also ensure that they have understood the information you have given them.

Documentation and record-keeping

You will be aware by now of the importance of documentation and record-keeping, which is integral to the care process. Consider the patient who has hand-held records. For example, if you are a midwife, your patient may have her own records. What happens if they are lost? Do you have a duplicated record of events recorded somewhere else? Some patients with chronic illness may also have hand-held records. It is vital here that you aware of local policy and Nursing and Midwifery Council guidelines for records and record-keeping (Nursing and Midwifery Council 2004).

Professional judgement and decision-making

What if the patient or their relatives are not happy about discharge? You may not feel that the patient is ready for discharge and, if so, how can you explain this? You may be given information by the patient or relative that raises questions about their readiness for discharge: what action will you take?

Risk management

Where does the framework of clinical governance sit with discharge planning? What can potentially go wrong? What might be the consequences of ineffective discharge?

Health care professionals must be able to recognise the abnormal as well as the normal.

Branches of discharge planning

These will be specific to the patient you have selected but you may have considered the following:

- Patient's physical status – activities of daily living including mobility, elimination, hygiene; does the patient need continuing support with this?
- Support in the community by formal/informal carers; inter-agency support may be required

- What continuing treatment is required? For example: medicines, pain relief, therapy, wound dressings, suture removal
- Psychological support – counselling, spiritual guidance
- Remember, patients will be discharged home to recover but some may also be discharged home to facilitate a peaceful death
- If a patient has undergone surgery, they must receive concise and appropriate advice about all sorts of matters from when can they eat normally to when can they drive their car
- Is a follow-up appointment required?

Now complete the tree from the perspective of another health care professional. If you are engaged on a programme that incorporates interprofessional learning, you could discuss this with a fellow student from the chosen discipline. Alternatively, if you are on placement you could liaise with a member of the multidisciplinary team to gain their perspective of their role and responsibilities.

Conclusions

Anyone wanting to work in health care settings will have to participate in multidisciplinary teamwork. Understanding what roles, goals and skills are involved is an essential part of any preparation for the work. Not only do you require skills to participate in teamwork but a team's culture will influence how you learn and develop skills for care. There is no getting away from teamwork, it's a fact of life in modern health care. If it is done well patients receive good care (Borill *et al.* 2001).

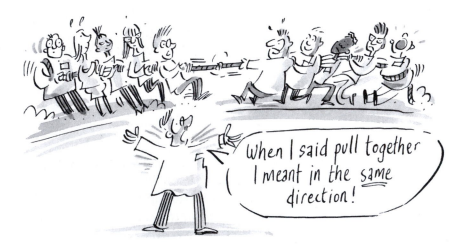

When I said pull together I meant in the *same* direction!

RRRRRRapid recap

Check your progress so far by working through each of the following questions.

1. List six characteristics of teams.
2. Why is discharge planning a major issue in health care?
3. Is your functional role the same as your team role?

If you have difficulty with more than one of the questions, read through the section again to refresh your understanding before moving on.

References

Bandura, A. (1977) *Social Learning Theory*. Prentice-Hall, Englewood Cliffs, NJ.

Belbin, M. (1993) *Team Roles at Work*. Butterworth-Heinemann, Oxford.

Borill, C., West, M., Dawson, J. *et al.* (2001) *Team Working and Effectiveness in Health Care. Findings from the Health Care Team Effectiveness Project*. Aston Business School, University of Leeds, Universities of Glasgow and Edinburgh, University of Sheffield. Available on line at: http://research.abs.aston.ac.uk/achsor/effectiveness.pdf.

Daly, J., Speedy, S., Jackson, D. and Darbyshire, P. (2002) *Contexts of Nursing: An introduction*. Blackwell, Oxford.

Department of Health (2000a) *The NHS Plan*. HMSO, London.

Department of Health (2000b) *Organisation with a Memory*. The Stationery Office, London.

Glen, S. and Leiba, T. (2002) *Multi-professional Learning for Nurses: Breaking the boundaries*. Palgrave Macmillan, Basingstoke.

Hornby, S. and Atkins, J. (2000) *Collaborative Care: Interprofessional, interagency and interpersonal*, 2nd edn. Blackwell Science, Oxford.

Howkins, E. and Thornton, C. (2002) *Managing and Leading Innovation in Health Care.* Baillière Tindall, London.

Mohram, S.A., Cohen, S.G. and Mohram, A.M. Jr (1995) *Designing Team Based Organizations*. Jossey-Bass, San Francisco, CA.

NHS Modernisation Agency (2004) *Series 3 Improvement Leaders Guide to Building and Nurturing an Improvement Culture*. Modernisation Agency, London.

Nursing and Midwifery Council (2002) *Code of Professional Conduct*. Nursing and Midwifery Council, London.

Nursing and Midwifery Council (2004) *Guidelines for Records and Record Keeping*. Nursing and Midwifery Council, London.

Vygotsky, L.S. (1978) *Mind in Society*. Harvard University Press, Cambridge, MA.

Walsh, M. and Walsh, A. (1998) Practice development units: a study of teamwork. *Nursing Standard*, **12**(33), 35–38.

Walsh, M. (2001) *Nursing Frontiers: Accountability and the boundaries of care*. Butterworth-Heinemann, Oxford.

Further reading

Buchanan, D. and Huczynski, A. (1997) *Organisational Behaviour: An introductory text*, 3rd edn. Prentice-Hall, Englewood Cliffs, NJ.

Northcott, N. (2003) Working within a health care team. In: Hinchliff, S., Norman, S. and Schober, J. (eds) *Nursing Practice and Health Care*, 4th edn. Edward Arnold, London.

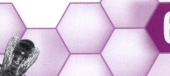

6

Learning, practice and policy

Learning outcomes

By the end of this chapter you should be able to:

- Understand the importance of continuing professional development and lifelong learning
- Use the Meaningful Assimilation of Skills for Care model to assist in personal and practice development
- Discuss how policy impacts on health care
- Identify the key documents in the modernisation agenda.

Introduction

You will not be developing your clinical skills in splendid isolation, nor will you be able to develop a range of skills solely because you want to. Your skills base will be determined by the requirements of the service users you work with – patients, carers, families – and the employer you work for. They will also be determined by the occupational group and/or professional regulatory body you are affiliated to. Your personal interest in developing skills does play a part in this equation but it will always be in competition with, or have to be prioritised against, the other power bases/stakeholders.

Power bases/stakeholders in skills development:

- Patient/service users' requirements
- Employer
- Regulatory body
- Own personal interest.

Using the MASC model and continuing to use the analogy of a tree we can develop the discussion surrounding these power bases and the influence they exert on skills development.

Growth and development

The leaves, branches and trunk of a tree are visible, tangible and attractive. When you first participate in care delivery you see discrete components of care (e.g. wound management, administration of medication, nutritional support) in the same way. Being involved in these activities is appealing. It involves direct patient contact and you feel that you are 'doing' something – it's tangible. You can make a real contribution to patient care that is visible to you and to others, such as patients and supervisors. It is in these early stages of development that you feel the need to focus on the psychomotor or task element of a skill. You need to find some way to articulate what you can and cannot do and identify where and how you will learn more.

This is the point at which you might choose to use the template from the MASC model. You would be able to identify and address all the obvious elements of a skill and some of the evidence base for practice. However in the longer term it would be the equivalent of appreciating the leaves, branches and trunk of a tree just for the appearance. This approach would ignore the complexity of cell structures, the chemistry and the symbiosis that occurs between the tree and its environment (see Chapter 4).

Some people will always appreciate a tree for its appearance alone (superficial); others will make the effort to understand how it functions (meaningful). You need to make a choice – are you going to leave your skills development at a superficial level or make it more meaningful? Some people abandon their skills development at this (template) stage. For example, they know how many chest compressions are required, at what depth and what speed, for cardiopulmonary resuscitation (CPR). They become comfortable. They have built up a level of proficiency in terms of the psychomotor element of their skills and know a little of the knowledge that relates to practice. Often the next stage of development – involving ethics, policy, organisational culture – is hard to 'see'. It involves the 'grey' areas of practice, so these people decide that it could be uncomfortable to go any further. This next stage of development involves managing uncertainty. In these circumstances your instinct will be to make sense of what you are experiencing by imposing some order on the uncertainly. We think that part of that process involves mapping and studying the roots and enablers of the MASC model.

A tree's roots are not instantly visible but must be present to allow the tree to grow. The viability and growth of your care skills depend on how well you attend to the roots of those skills, for example ensuring that you attend an annual update for CPR and deciding that you will attend advanced life support training. You're addressing the need for up-to-date *evidence* on which to base practice, maintaining your *professional* obligation to practise safely and have a *personal* interest in the skill, as you are applying for a post on a cardiology ward.

A tree's chances of survival will also depend on the interaction between environmental factors and the tree's internal systems and structures, such as photosynthesis. This is why we think the enablers are important in the MASC model. You can have the most proficient CPR skills on the cardiology ward because you have attended the update and training. The roots of CPR have been addressed, but you will not get the best clinical outcome for the patient or their family if you are brusque or distant while talking to them about the option of having a 'Do Not Resuscitate' request added to the patient's notes. You may be communicating in a defensive manner because you are unsure of your feelings on this subject, or how to cope with the feelings of the patient and their family if they are angry, they start to cry, or both. You need to have identified and developed the enablers linked to service-user involvement, emotional intelligence and interpersonal communication. Experiences such as this could lead to dissatisfaction with your performance and in turn make your working environment stressful; or alternatively they might stimulate the desire to learn more about the skills where you have a deficit.

You need to start thinking about the less tangible, less accessible and less obvious parts of skills development because they are no less important than the visible parts of care skills. If you are going to deliver holistic care then you need to be holistic in terms of your skills development. That means using all the parts of the MASC model for skills development – template, enablers and roots.

Growth – do you have a choice?

Earlier we asked if you were going to be happy to leave your care skills at a comfortable but superficial stage of development. We hope that answer was a resounding 'no'. We will now provide you with more reasons why growth and development are not optional; it's not a question of 'if', but to what extent.

What encourages a tree's growth? What nutrients are required in the soil, from where will it access water and how much light will it require to flourish? These are all the *extrinsic* factors that will affect the tree. When you are developing skills, some of the extrinsic factors that you require might include a safe environment in which to learn and work, having the correct life–work balance for your circumstances and being rewarded for the work you do. *Improving Working Lives* (Department of Health 2000a) addresses these issues and is one of the pillars of the Department of Health's human resources framework.

Your contribution to the care environment will be governed by membership of a professional body or occupational group. This will give you a sense of identity and initial sense of stability. Quite quickly you are socialised into the group's culture and reference to any standard sociology text book will provide an example of that process. Membership of that culture will also root your skills and knowledge in a particular niche. An initial tap root (pre-registration preparation) keeps developing until it becomes wide and deep and develops additional side roots; in the same way your evidence base and experiential knowledge should allow you to develop a network of skills and knowledge that go beyond what you first required.

Roots are flexible and allow for continuous growth and development – Continuing Professional Development (CPD). The MASC model should challenge you to include a wide range of evidence when developing your care skills; so wide in fact that you never stop learning, even when you've achieved a significant level of expertise. Once you are an expert you will be in a position to help and support others with their skills development. All of us want to achieve mastery and expertise in relation to the skills we use in care delivery. It gives us a sense of pride and satisfaction with the quality of the care we deliver.

As nurses we are regulated by the requirements of the Nursing and Midwifery Council (NMC) in relation to continuing professional development and lifelong learning. The NMC states that lifelong learning is: 'more than simply keeping up to date. It requires an enquiring approach to the practice of nursing and midwifery, as well as issues which impact on that practice' (Nursing and Midwifery Council 2002a, p. 3).

The professional obligation to embrace lifelong learning is reiterated, from an employers perspective, in *Working Together, Learning Together* (Department of Health 2001a), the lifelong learning strategy for the NHS. Some of the key characteristics of this strategy include your ability to understand the impact of constant change on the context of practice, be proactive and take responsibility for your own learning, and recognise future areas for personal and professional development. The word 'context' again bringing us back to the MASC model and emphasising the need for you to understand the setting in which you practise – get to know and understand your environment, don't just experience it.

There are many species of tree and they exist in a variety of environments. They adapt to the environment they grow in. Some like extremes, some like temperate climates. Similarly, there are a variety of clinical **ecosystems** with environments that you could find more or less comfortable to work in depending on your perspective. You could think that a coronary care unit was an extreme environment and a general surgical ward was a comfortable one. However a peer or colleague could believe the opposite to be true. Always try to remember that comfort is a commodity we need in a specific amount – not enough and we don't develop at all; too

○━┱ *Keywords*

Ecosystem

The plants and animals found in a specific location, which will react and adapt to the geographical, geological and weather conditions local to that area.

much and we can become complacent. You must also recognise that you are part of the system too. Clinical teams, wards or departments can be thought of as ecosystems or, as the NHS Modernisation Agency (2004a, p. 10) suggest, a 'clinical microsystem', i.e. the basic working unit for all care. An important feature of working in a team is that it can be challenging but can also help us cope with the stresses and strains of practice and lead to the opportunity to develop new skills. (For more details on teamwork see Chapter 5.)

Reflective activity

Have you ever studied or worked in an environment in which you felt uncomfortable? Why it was uncomfortable?
List the ways and means that you used to change the situation.
How many of these strategies did you control and how many were controlled by other people?

Complexity and constant change are features of all ecosystems and environments. A tree, like all living things, is designed to grow, move and adapt to change – so are we, it's part of our hard-wiring, it is intrinsic. Therefore we advocate that a love of learning, throughout life, should be intrinsic to all health care workers. The MASC model facilitates this in terms of skills development and mastery. It will help you to articulate all parts of that development:

- A rationale for choosing skills
- A way of focusing how to develop the skill
- A way to reflect and evaluate your performance.

This will include not only the obvious and easy to articulate components of care but the unseen more ethereal parts. You need to adapt to the demands placed on your skills and knowledge owing to the complexity and constant change of modern clinical environments. Using the MASC model regularly will ensure that you stay up to date.

When developing skills, understanding how that environment is organised and regulated is essential. There are a variety of documents used to communicate organisational and regulatory requirements, such as guidelines, legislation, standards for practice and expert opinion. It is also important to understand how each of the power bases/stakeholders influences the skills and care agenda by using **policy**. You need to understand not only how policy is formulated but also where and how you might play a role in its implementation and evaluation.

Keywords

Policy
A plan of action designed to ensure that an organisation runs smoothly. Several interested parties, e.g employers, customers, politicians, professionals, may play a part in the planning, implementation and evaluation of the policy.

Delivering care – policy and modernisation

From our experience of working with students the word 'policy' has been known to have a sedative effect. We think policy is such an important part of what shapes your clinical skills that you need to have an appreciation of it as a subject area. To make 'policy' a little more practical, and as an incentive for you to read this chapter completely, we want you to complete the next 'Over to you' before reading any further. Our aim is to prove to you that following a simple analysis of a problem you will be able to identify the interested parties and start to think about the processes policy-makers would use.

Over to you

Choose one of the following scenarios and decide how you would deal with the situation if you were in charge.

- You are the senior nurse in an A&E department. A new multi-million-pound bypass opened on the outskirts of town 6 months ago. There has been an 20% increase in the number of road traffic accidents in the past 4 months, all generated by two particular junctions on the bypass. The police, ambulance and fire services are worried about his trend.

Or:

- You are a hospital manager who has to oversee the closure of children's services at the local general hospital and transfer them to a city teaching hospital 20 miles away. The local newspaper has started a campaign to keep the services as they are. You have to move them because latest recommendations for safe practice insists that suitably qualified medical and nursing staff care for the children.

You need to know:

- Who will get involved
- What role the media would play
- What role there would be for local and national politicians/government
- What data and evidence you need
- How you will present your new ideas to the public
- How you will make changes; who will implement them
- Who will fund them
- How you will know if the improvement has worked.

Now that you have completed this exercise it should become apparent that policy will impact on you as a citizen as well as in your role of health care worker or student. Every activity that we are involved in – tourism, food production, education, transport – is shaped by policy. We hope we have convinced you to read the rest of this chapter, as well as the further reading listed at the end of the chapter. By doing this you will be able to identify specific examples of how policy has changed the delivery of care and in turn how this has required changes in staff education and skills development.

Policy – the impact

'Doing the right things at the right time for the right people, and doing them right – first time' (Department of Health 1997) sounds eminently sensible and the simplicity of the statement belies the complexity of what it involves. From a nursing perspective it would involve having the correct number of generalists and specialists, with a range of skills and a sound evidence base for practice, delivering care safely and effectively. So skills and knowledge sit at the heart of the policy agenda. The nursing profession has always spent time and energy ensuring that relevant skills were taught to its members so that they were capable of caring for the sick and the healthy. However, the set of skills required to be a nurse has never remained completely static. It changes over time as technology develops and roles are moved between occupation groups. The best possible formula for learning skills and choosing which skills should be learned is often debated among nurses, particularly between different generations of nurse (e.g. SRN, RGN, RN), as well as among politicians and the general public.

> ### Over to you
>
> Find newspaper articles about what people think of modern nursing and/or health care.
> How often do they refer to 'the good old days'?
> What skills do they suggest that nurses/health care workers need?
> Does that image fit with the requirements and demands of modern practice?

During the last 10 years there has been an increasing emphasis on learning skills for practice (e.g. Peach 1999). It has seemed as if nursing as a profession was on a quest for the Holy Grail of skills, education and development. The profession has gone through a seesaw experience similar to that mentioned in Chapter 3. The older style of apprenticeship training concentrated on tasks and the psychomotor element of care. Project 2000 produced nurses with enhanced communications skills and an appreciation of psychology and sociology but the public and the profession worried about their clinical skills at the point of registration. Now, with curricula based on the requirements of *Making a Difference* (Department of Health 1999a), we are in a situation where the 21st-century practitioner is prepared 50% of the time in a clinical practice setting and 50% of the time at university. This example of the changes in nurse education highlights how powerful policy can be. We would suggest that policy has a role in the unseen part of practice. It can be classified using roots and enablers in the MASC model. You will not escape feeling the impact of policy on practice and skills development, regardless of how many degrees of separation you think there may be between yourself and the policy makers.

The sense of separation is worth considering in a little more detail at this point. For many nurses the development of policy can seem very distant from their day to day experience of care delivery. Policy is something that politicians, civil servants, experts and senior managers formulate. Charities, pressure groups, professional lobbyists and the media may try to influence the choice of subject, the developmental phase of the process and the final outcome. Often they are working as advocates for service users. So the whole process involves a series of stakeholders trying to gain control over resources and how they are deployed, or influencing the way something is regulated.

Over to you

For a more comprehensive account of these issues, read Hennessy, D. and Spurgeon, P. (2000) Health Policy and Nursing: Influence, Development and Impact. Macmillan, Basingstoke.

Hennessy (2000, p. 3) cite Percival (1997), who sums up the roles nurses can have in relation to policy: 'They drive, they navigate, they repair faults, they lubricate the engine, but they do not often design new engines'. This may leave us with a sense of being an invaluable but small cog in a very large machine. We spend a lot of time implementing policy. That leaves us with a challenge as nurses – to get involved in setting the agenda before and during as well as after the policy is formulated. We have an opportunity to do just that through consultation with the policy-makers.

A good example of consultation with the public and staff was *Choice, Responsiveness and Equity in the NHS* (Department of Health 2003a).

The government was interested to know what changes would result in the greatest impact/improvement for patients, carers and

Over to you

Results from the *Choice, Responsiveness and Equity* consultation can be found in *Building on the Best* (Department of Health 2003b).

users. There was a particular emphasis on areas such as primary, emergency and planned care. Maternity care, children's health, mental health, continuing long-term conditions and care for older people were also included. As Maddock (2002) noted, the stakeholders in the modernisation process include 'practitioners, staff and users'. So as stakeholders it is in our own interest to be proactive and contribute to consultations.

As nurses we also have a professional obligation to participate in policy development (Hennessy 2000), as we are concerned about the quality of the care we provide. We could be called upon to act as an advocate for patients/service users. They are not always in a position to speak out about concerns such as lack of information, being exposed to dangerous practice or being denied access to services. We need to be aware of organisational issues affecting care, such as inappropriate skill mix or delegation of care, and react to those circumstances professionally.

Over to you

Identify the clauses in the *Code of Professional Conduct* (Nursing and Midwifery Council 2002b), that you think are linked to the themes of:

● Information
● Managing risk
● Ensuring equality.

(Access the relevant code or standards for practice if this document does not apply to your professional background.)

So, to recap before we go any further, policy can seem a bit dry to begin with but there are important and practical reasons why it cannot be ignored. We have established that policy has brought about changes in nurse education and has therefore influenced the preparation and skills that nurses have. Various stakeholders will try to influence how policy is generated, implemented and evaluated. We are stakeholders depending on our various roles, as citizens, students, family members and care workers. As stakeholders we should be involved in all stages of the policy process, not only for personal reasons but as a professional obligation also.

Policy and skills

To further illustrate the potential that policy has to shape clinical environments and your skills development, we would now like to discuss two specific examples of policy – an Act of Parliament and a National Service Framework – and the impact they have had on skills.

The National Health Service and Community Care Act 1990 resulted in many patients moving from large institutional settings to small residential homes, or setting up their own home for the first time. Nurses who had always worked in large hospital settings found themselves in primary care settings. They had to develop the skills required of community nurses, for example understanding family dynamics and how they impact on decision-making; the different styles of interpersonal skill required once in the client's home; different styles of time management; how to maintain hand hygiene when there is no access to hot water, soap and hand towel. The introduction of the internal market brought with it the concept of patients as consumers or customers. *The Patients' Charter* (Department of Health 1991) and the requirement to have a 'named (qualified) nurse' also occurred around this time. This resulted in changes to nursing practice, particularly new communication skills. For example, nurses had to learn how to encourage patients and clients to provide feedback on the care they received, and if necessary how to access the complaints procedure. Junior staff nurses became named nurses and as such were given the opportunity to liaise with other members of the multidisciplinary team. In the past this would have been the role of the nurse in charge. The way that teams of practitioners worked together changed as a consequence, for example primary nursing (Wright 1994). Evidence-based practice was advocated as a way to improve care, resulting in information retrieval, change management and clinical audit skills being developed by all clinical staff.

Current examples of policy influencing skills development can be found in the National Service Frameworks, one of which relates specifically to coronary heart disease (Department of Health 2000b, c). Because of the requirements of the National Service Frameworks, specifically Standard 6, a patient with a heart attack needs to be assessed and given a specific type of medication 'within 60 minutes of calling for professional help'. This has resulted in qualified nurses who specialise in cardiac care developing their skills and knowledge to the point at which they are competent and confident enough to commence this treatment. It means that the patient is treated efficiently and effectively because the therapy is not delayed until a specific professional, i.e. a doctor, is available.

You may be able to find examples like this locally, where new roles have developed in relation to a specific area of practice (e.g. Clinical Nurse Specialist – Endoscopy, Nurse Practitioner – A&E). All these developments tend to have occurred as a result of policy, which is driving multidisciplinary teams to work in new ways.

Modernisation is a strong theme in current health policy documents such as *The NHS Plan* (Department of Health 2000d) and *The NHS Improvement Plan* (Department of Health 2004a). Government policy can be summed up as follows:

- The NHS has to be redesigned around the needs of the patient, who may be an expert in their own care
- There needs to be more, better paid staff, using new ways of working to deliver this service, with a clear career structure.

The patient's experience

One of the important things that we can do as health care workers is appreciate what it's like to be a patient/client accessing care. Many of us have been service users in our own right, or may have accompanied a family member or friend while they accessed health services. We can also appreciate that patients with chronic or long-term illness may in fact know more about the management of that illness than we do. This has been recognised by the publication of *The Expert Patient* (Department of Health 2002a).

Working with 'expert patients' will mean that staff have to change the way they see their role. In the past the care worker or professional was in charge; they often made most of the decisions in the care process, informing the patient but not necessarily involving them fully. Now the service user's opinion, participation and involvement is something that we all need to encourage as health care workers. For example 'support patient's choices' may mean that the patient hasn't chosen the option that you recommend but an equally safe alternative. This involves sound decision-making skills, the ability to manage risk, evidence-based practice and sophisticated interpersonal communication skills on your part. As a service user you would expect to be allowed to contribute fully in decisions about your care, so it's from a service user's perspective that we will continue this discussion.

əviɟɔəЯ**Reflective activity**

Think about your last visit to the dentist, GP or outpatients department, or an admission to hospital. What were the five most vivid memories you took away from the experience?

Regardless of the expertise of the patient, each individual will have to negotiate a particular pathway or process, from initial identification of a problem to investigations, treatment and recovery. The patient's journey can provide a series of complications beyond those of the injury or illness they have. As on any journey, the patient might feel they've been exposed to a foreign language (medical jargon), seen an interesting collection of health tribes, all dressed in their various clan colours (a multidisciplinary team), sat in traffic jams (reception, in- and outpatients department) and even suffered cancellations (surgery rescheduled). The whole experience can be overwhelming.

In the past the journey/process could be slowed down or even stalled for several reasons. Sometimes there were not enough staff. On other occasions the staff on duty didn't have the correct skills or knowledge to care for the patient. For instance, when all the members of a consultant surgeon's team were busy in theatre, A&E, outpatients, the intensive care unit and a variety of wards, this could leave one ward with no immediate medical care, unless there was an emergency such as a cardiac arrest. Of course, the medical staff could be paged, but they would have to prioritise the request from the ward with whatever they were doing at the time. If a patient required a new intravenous cannula and had signs and symptoms of a chest infection the nurses would have to wait for a doctor to come and re-site the cannula, sign the X-ray request and prescribe an antibiotic. If the doctor decided that other patients had a greater clinical need, this patient's care was delayed. It wasn't the case that the nurses didn't want to do these things but that legislation and organisational systems acted as barriers to the development and use of these skills. Many of these barriers have been removed, so the staff have new ways of working and the patient's journey is more straightforward.

Not only should the patient's journey through the health care system be as smooth as possible but it is sometimes worth considering how to redesign it. A process should not remain the same, particularly if it's not resulting in the best clinical outcome for the patient and if it's based on custom. The NHS Modernisation

Agency has published a series of Improvement Leader's Guides, one of which – *Process Mapping, Analysis and Redesign* (NHS Modernisation Agency 2002) – gives some concrete examples of how you can start to build a picture of the patient's experience, where you fit into the process and how redesigning services could involve practice development. One example is nurse-led clinics. Taking our example of the surgical ward, the improved process for the patient would mean that the nurse could perform a physical examination of their chest, request an X-ray and prescribe the first dose of antibiotics, resulting in faster and more efficient care. So its clear that what is required for the patient's journey to be redesigned is a simultaneous redesign of staff roles and staff development (Department of Health/Royal College of Nursing 2003).

The staff development agenda

When mapping the patient's journey, health care workers need to consider what skills are required to deliver care throughout that process. Then they have to decide if they have those skills – if so, then how do they maintain them; if not, how and where can they develop them? As we have already suggested, the skills that you have today will not mean that you are able or competent to practise in 5 years time (Nursing and Midwifery Council 2002b), especially with services being updated and reconfigured regularly and the evidence base for practice evolving continuously. The role that you eventually find yourself in may be very different from that which you expected to fill when you started your career.

This evolution in roles and skills development is something that can be tracked throughout history. At one time blood pressure measurement would have been deemed to be an activity only appropriate for medical staff or their students. It would have been at the cutting edge of technology. Now it's a very ordinary activity in any clinical environment. It is carried out, using a variety of techniques and equipment, by nurses, health care assistants, physiotherapists and podiatrists.

We sometimes equate roles with certain sets of skills and a specific knowledge base. For instance, doctors do 'this', physiotherapists do 'that'. Dietitians know about 'X', radiographers know about 'Y'. The situation that we find ourselves in today regarding skills and knowledge has a historical dimension, which goes beyond the evolutionary process we've just mentioned in relation to blood pressure.

History

Understanding the history of the occupational roles in today's health service helps us to understand our current situation, hopefully making it easier to see how we can move forward. In the UK we have a long history of education and training specifically for health professionals/workers. For example, St Thomas's nurse training school was set up in the 1860s (Dingwall *et al.* 1988).Each group of workers had a specific range of skills, usually prescribed by gender, class and level of education. Nurses were thought to be good at caring because they were women. They had no natural capacity for anything technical, such as science, diagnosis or performing surgery. Different skills carried different degrees of status. Washing and feeding patients, attending to bodily functions like elimination and dealing with body fluids, the work of nurses, was perceived as low-status because it was 'dirty' work. Alternatively, applying a dressing or taking a blood pressure measurement had higher status and was technical.

The impact of gender on knowledge and care are subjects you will need to read more about to fully understand skills development, interprofessional relationships and the status of care. See the further reading list for more information.

The legacy of the historical gender/care debate that we inherited as nurses was the stalled patient experience mentioned earlier and the resulting frustration we felt on a daily basis, not being able to develop skills because it was thought inappropriate for us to do so, by medical staff, politicians and sometimes colleagues. (Again the impact of policy was shaping practice.) There were professional boundaries and our skills were expected to stay within them. For many years nurses had developed experiential knowledge, which meant they could diagnose a range of conditions and prescribe medications appropriately. They could also decide when/if certain diagnostic tests were required. However this was outside the scope of their role. Organisational systems and legislation meant that they would have to wait for another health care professional to authorise these activities. For example, a doctor had to sign an X-ray request and to bring in a dietitian would require a formal referral from a doctor, even though the nurse had already discussed the potential referral with the doctor.

However the boundaries between health professionals are shifting, resulting in a shift in their skills development. Walsh (2000) discusses the variables influencing contemporary practice, why the shift has occurred and what the nursing profession will have to consider in terms of development and accountability. Key policy documents in the field of staff development include *A Health Service of all the Talents: Developing the NHS workforce.* (Department of Health 2000e) and *Shifting the Balance of Power: Securing delivery – human resources framework* (Department of Health 2001b).

Another reason why some nurses are developing skills and practising differently is a result of the working time directive, which was implemented in full in August 2004. The most noticeable result of the working time directive is the reduction in junior doctors' hours. Other members of staff are expected to develop their roles and skills to continue to deliver services at their current level in the absence of doctors. Many staff are experiencing role transition and in some cases role innovation – new roles will emerge, such as assistant practitioner and surgical practitioner. Examples of these roles can be found at European Working Time Directive FAQ (Department of Health 2004b).

Nurses do not want to be doctors, nor should they be forced to feel that that is the direction in which their profession is being driven. Many nurses are now gaining additional education and qualifications in skills such as physical examination, prescribing and ordering tests/investigations because it is appropriate to the environment they work in and the client group they work with. Nurse practitioners were one specific group who led this area of skills development. Walsh (1999) suggests that nurse practitioners were maxi nurses not mini doctors. Nurses should use and adopt medical skills to enhance the care they give patients but all the while retain a nurse's perspective. This type of role development is also found in the Chief Nursing Officer's ten key targets (Department of Health 2002b)

Although role and skills development has previously been ad hoc and based on local arrangements, the Skills Escalator (Department of Health 2003c) now provides a clear seven-step career structure. Using a variety of nursing roles we can apply the skills and knowledge related to nutritional care to steps 4, 5, 6 and 7 of the skills escalator (Table 6.1, pp. 154–155). We have also applied the some examples of role redesign identified by the NHS Modernisation Agency (2004b). We think it's worth noting that your career progression can be linear, i.e. you move up the escalator. However once you are a very senior member of staff you are often in situations where you might have to develop a depth or breadth of knowledge not currently expected of your occupational group. Or your role could be so innovative that you have to design it yourself!

Table 6.1 Applying skills to role development

Step on the escalator	Knowledge, skills and competence – nutrition
4. Cadet Nurse/Student Nurse NHS Modernisation Agency 2004b: Moving along a traditional skills ladder, both roles well established within nursing	• Understands anatomy and physiology of the digestive system; basic comprehension of some diseases that affect the system • Understands the components of a healthy diet • Knows how to order and access appropriate diets for patients • Can assist in the administration of medication • Can assist patients who have problems with eating and drinking • Can provide assistance with nasogastric (NG) feeds, percutaneous endoscopic gastrostomy (PEG) feeds and monitoring total parenteral nutrition (TPN) • Records dietary intake, implements care as prescribed and assist in evaluation • Can assist in nutritional screening
5. Registered Nurse NHS Modernisation Agency 2004b: Moving up a traditional skills ladder, another well established role within nursing but with obvious progress available within the same role	All the above and: • Intermediate knowledge of the gastrointestinal tract and altered physiology • Understands the components of a healthy diet and is aware of health promotion models and techniques • Understands the requirements of clinical nutrition and techniques used to provided for nutritional support – NG, PEG, TPN • Administers medication • Can assess, plan, implement and evaluate • Can send appropriate referral to dietetics department • Can support patients who have difficulty swallowing and those with altered body image, taking into account the psychosocial dimensions of nutrition • Can insert a nasogastric tube, can change TPN infusions • Is aware of and knows how to implement local health and safety policies in relation to food handling and ensures that other members of staff comply • Participates in the audit process
6. Ward Manager/Sister/Charge Nurse or Clinical Nurse Specialist – Nutrition NHS Modernisation Agency 2004b: Expanding in breadth and or depth of role i Ward manager's role is traditional but there have been developments in the breadth of the role such as 24-hour management responsibility and financial accountability ii Clinical Nurse Specialist will have a deep knowledge base and matching skills	All the above and: • Leadership role within a clinical team – advanced interpersonal skills, e.g. holds a counselling qualification • Provides education for staff, patients and carers • Has control over resources, e.g. budgets/equipment, staffing • Advanced clinical skills, e.g. physical examination, chest percussion, can prescribe, can order diagnostic tests, admit and discharge patients • Maintains standards of care, e.g. *Essence of Care* benchmarks, designs, audits • Clinical Nurse Specialist may work in primary and secondary health care settings

Table 6.1 *continued*	
7. Nurse consultant NHS Modernisation Agency 2004b: New role. At senior levels, staff will have to work with very broad job descriptions and shape new role so that it is appropriate to the environment or organisation they work in	All the above and: ● Has own case load, admits, plans, implements and evaluates care and discharges own patients ● Finds funding for own research and designs methodology; coordinates the data collection and analysis ● Is responsible for dissemination of results and ensuring that they are used in practice ● Teaching links with local university, teaches across academic levels ● Liaises with Trust Board, Royal College of Nursing, Department of Health – develops policy and strategy

We are making no claims of absolute accuracy regarding the skills and knowledge described at each stage. They are presented primarily to illustrate a sense of progression from novice to expert (Benner 1984). To find examples of how roles are being developed at each step of the escalator you can access the Department of Health's web site, www.dh.gov.uk, and then follow the links through Policy and guidance, Human resources and training and Model career until you reach the link for the Skills Escalator.

Skills matter

Hopefully, you are still with us and are becoming more comfortable thinking about policy in relation to practice. Having established links between the patient's experience of the care system, service design and staff development, we have yet another example of how policy relates to the skills required to provide care. It could provide you with the strongest motivation yet to develop an interest in policy.

The opportunities to provide high-quality care, work hard and have a happy home life, participate fully as a member of a team and develop skills and access education and training are all rewarding. That's what attracts people to work in health care. Rewards are essential to our self-esteem and personal identity. Rewards can be social, such as being held in high regard by your family and neighbours because you do a worthwhile job. You could find your role personally rewarding because you enjoy helping people and believe that your work contributes to a healthier nation. There is one reward system that we haven't mentioned yet – pay.

The *Agenda for Change* pay structure (Department of Health 1999b) is due to be adopted throughout the NHS and the Department of Health expects all staff to be using the system by September 2005 (Department of Health 2004c). Excluding doctors and dentists and some managers, all staff will be using this system and, considering that there are one million NHS employees in

England alone (Department of Health 2001a), this is a major event. Although we acknowledge that many of you reading this book will work outside the NHS, it is such a large organisation that any change inside the NHS tends to have a ripple effect on other health care providers in the UK, so that is our rationale for discussing *Agenda for Change* further.

Implementation of the new pay structure is going to require job evaluation. That will involve measuring your 'job-related skills, knowledge and responsibilities' (Department of Health 2004c) so that you can be allocated an appropriate place on the relevant pay spine. Implementation will also utilise the Knowledge and Skills Framework (Department of Health 2003d), which is designed to:

- Identify the knowledge and skills that individuals need to *apply* [their emphasis] in their post
- Help guide the development of individuals
- Provided a fair and objective framework on which to base review and development for all staff
- Provide the basis of pay progression for all staff.

Taking a closer look at the Knowledge and Skills Framework it is interesting to see the links being made between skills, knowledge and the requirement to keep developing practice. This takes us back to our earlier arguments about growth, lifelong learning and continuing professional development. It's an example of how one of the power bases/stakeholders – the Department of Health/employer – is really making their present felt. 'Development review' will occur annually for NHS employees, resulting in a personal development plan. The Department of Health (2003d) suggests that this process is based on an adult learning cycle and cites the work of Kolb (1994). Again, we have advocated similar philosophies for your learning and development with the MASC model (Chapter 2). We would argue that our model is a good fit for contemporary practice and is compatible with many current policies.

In the past, nurses were quite reticent about discussing their skills and didn't always possess a vocabulary that could easily capture the complexity of what they did. We didn't often have to articulate what we did or what we knew because we were not asked to. If we did participate in these types of discussion it was with our peers, or students, and because they belonged to the same tribe they were used to the informal language and communication styles we used. For example, the translation of 'my gut instinct told me Jack would go off at tea time, that's why I had the trolley ready' is 'as an experienced respiratory nurse I could tell from Jack's vital signs, his wife's comments about him being restless and his increasing

confusion that there was potentially a serious problem developing.
I also knew the ward was about to become busy. That's why I placed
the resuscitation trolley around the corner from Jack's cubicle.'
(For more details about this phenomenon, see Chapter 3.) Because
we were not asked the question 'What skills do you use?', we didn't
tend to think about or rehearse the answer. This is not longer the
case. You are definitely going to be asked this question.

If you are involved in job evaluation, development review and
service and role redesign, it is clear that you will be asked to discuss
your skills. You will be required to articulate clearly, both verbally
and in writing:

- What your skills are
- How well you deliver these skills
- What skills you need to develop
- How you will find the correct support, training and education to
  do this.

You may have to present this material to a variety of audiences.
These audience will be affiliated to the stakeholders and power
bases we mentioned at the start of this chapter. All of them will be
interested in your competence to carry out the skills essential to
your occupational group and role. For example, in the case of the
NHS we've just highlighted the relationship that has been
established between articulating skills and knowledge development
and pay (Department of Health 1999b, 2004c). Professional and
regulatory bodies will also require evidence that you have the
appropriate skills and knowledge and have participated in
development of both, at the point of qualification and registration
and also as part of your continuing professional development (e.g.
Nursing and Midwifery Council 2002a).

You need to be able to explain your skills and knowledge to an
increasingly well informed population of service users, who need to
be seen as partners in their own care, not as passive recipients of
the ministrations of health care workers. Finally, for yourself, you
should be able to reflect on your own development and have an
awareness of your own practice that is based on evidence. This
should result in your being proactive about your skills development.

For instance, suppose you want to attend a 3-day course on de-
escalating aggression. You have used structured reflection to analyse
an incident from your latest clinical placement that provides
evidence that you need additional knowledge and an opportunity to
practise some communication techniques. You have rationalised that
there will be a positive outcome for the clinical area – you're
providing feedback and you will be in a stronger position to deal with

aggression so that it doesn't develop into violence, so improving the quality of care. This will make a strong case to present to a supervisor if there is a lot of competition for places on the course. It will also sound more professional than 'I want to go cos it might come in handy'.

We hope that by using the MASC model regularly you will develop the habit of articulating your skills and knowledge, the evidence base for practice and how you make sense of and understand care delivery. You will be rehearsing constantly, so that if you need to give a performance, i.e. answer questions about your skills, you will cope with any audience. Hopefully you can see some common ground between the MASC model and the professional and organisational systems that you will be expected to engage with. Benton (2003) suggests that education providers will have to support learning and development of skills rather than being purveyors of knowledge. We hope to do that with the MASC model – we are giving you a way to update continuously, not just highlighting the knowledge and processes involved in skills procedures. We hope that we have taught you to fish, as opposed to catching the fish for you.

Need

The skills and knowledge that you first discuss as part of an appraisal or personal development plan may seem basic. Over time they will become increasingly complex. It's like learning to fish in shallow waters, catching minnows. With experience you move into deeper water and the fish you catch are larger. Your confidence and motivation will develop incrementally as long as you feel safe. What you need at each stage of your development will be different (fishing rod, fishing net, fishing boat). To illustrate this point we have drawn some parallels with Maslow's hierarchy of needs, as described in Gross and McIlveen (1998). Maslow identified a hierarchy of needs, starting with basics like food and safety. Moving up the hierarchy he then identified psychological needs related to love, belonging and esteem. Finally, spiritual needs, or 'self-actualisation' – which is defined as 'a self initiated striving to become whatever we believe we are capable of being' (Gross and McIlveen 1998, p. 142) – top the hierarchy. Maslow suggested that we must have the most basic needs met before we can consider addressing our psychological or spiritual needs. We believe that you need to attend to the basic components of skills in the early stages of your development before you can progress to the more sophisticated element of care – for example contextual, professional.

Let's take recording a patient's temperature as an example.

- **Basic needs** – first-year Student Nurse. You will have to under-stand health and safety issues related to the appropriate use of equipment, how and where to place a thermometer (psychomotor/basic component) and the biology of circadian rhythms in relation to the most useful times of day to record temperature. You're involved in recording a patient's temperature because it has been delegated to you by a supervisor, e.g. your mentor. You have to perform safely and responsibly because you are contracted to work to specific levels of performance, often being assessed before you can progress to the next level of the skill.

- **Intermediate needs** – newly qualified Staff Nurse. You have mastery of taking and recording temperatures. You understand why temperature is a useful screening tool for diagnosing infection. With time and experience you may be managing a ward team, caring for 30 patients. Not only do you understand the psychomotor part of the skill, you are also conscious of the importance of correct delegation of this work, how it should not be carried out routinely but on an individual basis related to the patient's condition. Your needs at this stage could be learning how to delegate work without offending team members, yet remaining assertive, learning how to manage conflict and the need to put the theory of accountability into practice. Part of your motivation now relates to your continuing professional development and you access a short course in health-care-acquired infection.

- **Complex needs** – Sister. You still know how to measure and record a patient's temperature, but don't have to practise the skill very often. You will have to decide how proficient other members of staff are when they record temperature and you'll decide what training is on offer for staff such as cadets or health care assistants. You know the specification and cost of a variety of thermometers and will have to a carry out a cost–benefit analysis of several models to determine which is the best buy. You have mastered resource management skills such as delegation. You understand the knowledge underpinning infection control. You can practise holistically, taking a patient's physical, psychological and spiritual need into account while providing care. You can also provide care for the patient's family, either by providing information at first hand or by supporting staff nurses while they carry out that role. Your needs at this stage may link to team building strategies, learning how to chair meetings and participate in board meetings.

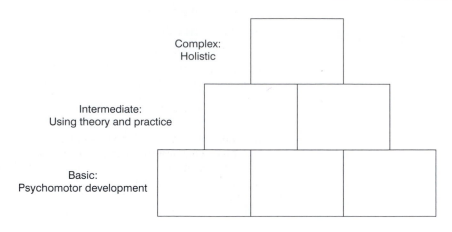

Figure 6.1 *Development needs.*

The basic needs are the building blocks for the intermediate level of practice, which in turn provide a base for the complex level of practice. You can't make progress unless you have mastery of the level at which you currently practise.

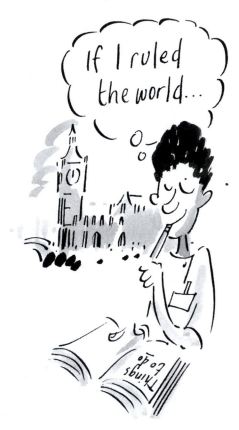

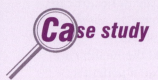

Case study

Malcolm's appointment – potential for role and skills development

Malcolm Stewart is a 74-year-old retired bus driver. He has had lower back pain for 2 years and is starting to get shooting pains down the back of his left leg, including short episodes of pins and needles. He is finding it difficult to walk, sit or stand for any length of time. He has not been able to sleep properly for the past 3 months and is worried and fed up. Following a visit to his GP, he has been referred to the orthopaedic clinic at his local hospital. He is with his daughter Theresa.

Theresa and Malcolm arrive at the hospital early so they can find a parking place. Malcolm gives his details to the receptionist and confirms the time of his appointment. Twenty minutes after his scheduled appointment he is called to sit in a consulting room. A health care assistant checks his weight, height and vital signs. She also asks him to provide a urine sample, gives him a receptacle and shows him where the toilets are. Once he has provided the sample, the nurse asks him to sit back in the consulting room. Ten minutes later the doctor arrives, takes Malcolm's medical history and performs a physical examination. Because of his pain it is difficult for Malcolm to get on to the examination couch. The doctor asks other members of a staff to provide Malcolm with assistance. Malcolm requires an X-ray. The X-ray department is on another floor and quite a distance away. Theresa asks the nurse if they can have a wheelchair to get there. The nurse arranges this with a porter. Once again, Malcolm has to present the request for the X-ray and confirm his details at a reception desk, and waits 10 minutes. When he gets back to outpatients he is led to a different room and a different nurse takes a blood sample . . .

Over to you

Although we haven't given you the full account of Malcolm's trip to hospital, try to answer the following questions:

- How would you improve Malcolm's experience of the Outpatients Department?
- How many of these improvements would involve the staff developing their roles/skills?
- How would you redesign this department so that it was more user friendly?

Conclusion

In order to consider your ongoing development needs, you need to acknowledge that the clinical environment is controlled and influenced by employers, professionals and patients. Your personal requirements are constantly merging and competing with these three power bases. Policy is formulated from the contribution of all three groups. You may belong to one or all of them at any given time, so you should be involved in more than implementation of policy.

As policy can bring about change on a massive scale in health care, impacting directly on your practice, it is wise to have an appreciation of the policy process and how and where to access policy documents. Throughout history policy has shaped the health care system we have now and that in turn has produced a patient's experience of care that can be difficult at times and sometimes needs to be redesigned. In redesigning the patient's experience we need to redesign our role and therefore develop our skills in ways that were not thought possible in the past because of role boundaries.

We propose the MASC model as a way for you to articulate the seen and unseen components of skills development, over time and taking many of the variables of the clinical environment into account, for training needs analysis, continuing professional development or to ensure correct placement on a pay spine. However, its primary purpose is to facilitate confident, competent and appropriate skills development as a way of ensuring high-quality patient-focused care.

RRRRRR*Rapid recap*

Check your progress so far by working through each of the following questions.

1. Where can you find policy documents?
2. How might you summarise the government's modernisation agenda?
3. How would you identify the skills and knowledge associated with your role?
4. How would you define lifelong learning?

If you have difficulty with more than one of the questions, read through the section again to refresh your understanding before moving on.

References

Benner, P. (1984) *From Novice to Expert: Excellence and power in clinical nursing practice*. Addison-Wesley, Menlo Park, CA.

Benton, D. (2003) Agenda for change: job evaluation. *Nursing Standard*, **17**(36), 39.

Department of Health (1991) *The Patient's Charter – Raising standards*. HMSO, London.

Department of Health (1997) *The New NHS – Modern, dependable. Cmd 3807*. HMSO, London. Available on line at: www.archive.official-documents.co.uk/documents/doh/newnhs.htm (last accessed 19.10.04).

Department of Health (1999a) *Making a Difference: Strengthening the nursing, midwifery and health visiting contribution to health and health care – summary*. Department of Health, London. Available on line at: www.dh.gov.uk/assetRoot/04/04/28/71/04042871.pdf (last accessed 19.10.04).

Department of Health (1999b) *Agenda for Change – Modernising the NHS pay system*. Department of Health, London. Available on line at: www.doh.gov.uk/agendaforchange/agenda.htm (last accessed 31.7.01).

Department of Health (2000a) *Improving Working Lives in the NHS*. Department of Health, London. Available on line at: www.dh.gov.uk/assetRoot/04/07/40/65/04074065.pdf (last accessed 19.10.04).

Department of Health (2000b) *National Service Framework for Coronary Heart Disease*. Department of Health, London. Available on line at: www.dh.gov.uk/assetRoot/04/04/90/70/04049070.pdf (last accessed 19.10.04).

Department of Health (2000c) *Getting the Right Skills to Deliver the CHD NSF – A guide for meeting workforce need*. Department of Health, London. Available on line at: www.dh.go.uk/PolicyAndGidance/HealthAndSocailCareTopics (last accessed 19.10.04).

Department of Health (2000d) *NHS Plan. A plan for investment, a plan for reform – a summary*. Department of Health, London. Available on line at: www.dh.gov/assetRoot/04/05/58/63/04055863.pdf (last accessed 19.10.04).

Department of Health (2000e) *A Health Service of all the Talents: Developing the NHS Workforce. Consultation document on the review of workforce planning*. Department of Health, London. Available on line at: www.dh.gov.uk/assetRoot/04/08/02/58/0408025.pdf (last accessed 19.7.04).

Department of Health (2001a) *Working Together, Learning Together – A framework for lifelong learning for the NHS*. Department of Health, London. Available on line at: www.dh.gov.uk/assetRoot/04/05/88/96/04058896.pdf (last accessed 19.10.04).

Department of Health (2001b) *Shifting the Balance of Power: Securing delivery – human resources framework*. Department of Health, London.

Department of Health (2002a) *The Expert Patient: A new approach to chronic disease management for the 21st century*. Department of Health, London. Available on line at: www.dh.gov.uk/assetRoot/04/01/85/78/04018578.pdf (last accessed 19.10.04).

Department of Health (2002b) *Developing Key Roles for Nurses and Midwives: A guide for managers*. Department of Health, London.

Department of Health (2003a) *Choice, Responsiveness and Equity in the NHS and Social Care: A national consultation. Resource Pack*. Department of Health, London.

Department of Health (2003b) *Building on the Best: Choice, responsiveness and equity in the NHS – a summary*. Department of Health, London. Available on line at: www.dh.gov.uk/assetRoot/04/07/52/99/04075299.pdf (last accessed 19.10.04).

Department of Health (2003c) *Illustrative Categories of Development within the Skills Escalator*. Department of Health, London. Available on line at: www.doh.gov.uk/hrinthenhs/learning/section4b/Secategoriesmenu.htm (last accessed 20.10.03).

Department of Health (2003d) *The NHS Knowledge and Skills Framework and Related Development Review*. Version 6, Working Draft. Department of Health, London.

Department of Health (2004a) *The NHS Improvement Plan: Putting people at the heart of public services. Executive summary*. Department of Health, London. Available on line at: www.dh.gov.uk/assetRoot/04/08/45/23/04084523.pdf (last accessed 19.10.04).

Department of Health (2004b) *European Working Time Directive FAQ*. Department of Health, London. Available on line at: www.dh.gov.uk/Policy and Guidance/HumanResourcesAnd Training/WorkingTimeDirective (last accessed 12.7.04).

Department of Health (2004c) *Agenda for Change: What will it mean for you? A guide for staff*. Department of Health, London. Available on line at: www.dh.gov/asetRoot/04/09/08/59 (last accessed 19.10.04).

Department of Health/Royal College of Nursing (2003) *Freedom to Practice: Dispelling the myths*. Department of Health, London.

Dingwall, R., Rafferty, A.M. and Webster, C. (1988) *An Introduction to the Social History of Nursing*. Routledge, London.

Gross, R. and McIlveen, R. (1998) *Psychology: A new introduction*. Hodder & Stoughton, London.

Hennessy, D. (2000) Chapter One The Emerging Themes pp. 1–38. In: Hennessy, D. and Spurgeon, P. *Health Policy and Nursing: Influence, development and impact*. Macmillan, Basingstoke.

Hennessy, D. and Spurgeon, P. (2000) *Health Policy and Nursing: Influence, development and impact*. Macmillan, Basingstoke.

Kolb, D. (1994) *Experiential Learning: Experiences as a source of learning and development*. Prentice Hall, Englewood Cliffs, NJ.

Maddock, S. (2002) Making modernisation work: new narratives change strategies and people management in the public sector. *International Journal of Public Sector Management*, **15**, 13–43.

National Health Service and Community Care Act 1990. HMSO, London.

NHS Modernisation Agency (2002) *Improvement Leaders' Guide to Process Mapping, Analysis and Redesign*. NHS Modernisation Agency, London.

NHS Modernisation Agency (2004a) *Improvement Leaders' Guide to Building and Nurturing an Improvement Culture*. Series 3. NHS Modernisation Agency, London.

NHS Modernisation Agency (2004b) *Improvement Leaders' Guide to Redesigning Roles*. Series 3. NHS Modernisation Agency, London.

Nursing and Midwifery Council (2002a) *Supporting Nurses and Midwives Through Life Long Learning*. Nursing and Midwifery Council, London.

Nursing and Midwifery Council (2002b) *Code of Professional Conduct*. Nursing and Midwifery Council, London.

Peach, L. (1999) *Fitness for Practice*. The UKCC Commission for Nursing and Midwifery Education. United Kingdom Central Council, London.

Walsh, M. (1999) Nurses and Nurse Practitioners: priorities in care. *Nursing Standard*, **13**(24), 38–42.

Walsh, M. (2000) *Nursing Frontiers: Accountability and boundaries of care*. Butterworth-Heinemann, Oxford.

Wright, S.G. (1994) *My Patient – My Nurse: The practice of primary nursing*, 2nd edn. Scutari Press, London.

Further reading

Allen, D. and Hughes, D. (2002) *Nursing and the Division of Labour in Healthcare*. Palgrave Macmillan, Basingstoke.

Department of Health (2003) *Delivering the HR in the NHS Plan – 2003*. Department of Health, London.

Lawler, J. (1991) *Behind the Screens*. Churchill Livingstone, Edinburgh.

McKay, L. (1993) *Conflicts in Care Medicine and Nursing*. Chapman & Hall, London.

Malin, N., Wilmot, S. and Manthorpe, J. (2002) *Key Concepts and Debates in Health and Social Policy*. Open University Press, Buckingham.

Soothill, K., Henry, C. and Kendrick, K. (1996) *Themes and Perspectives in Nursing*, 2nd edn. Chapman & Hall, London.

Appendix A

Rapid recap – answers

Chapter 1

1. What 'key' skills do you need to draw on to deliver individualised and holistic care?

1. Verbal and non-verbal communication

 Interpersonal skills

 Assessment

 Observation

 Interpretation

 Decision-making

 Respect and thoughtfulness.

2. What knowledge and understanding do you need to 'perform' a skill to an acceptable standard that ensures patient safety, comfort and dignity?

2. Underpinning theory

 Evidence base for practice

 Patient factors

 Clinical context

 Trust policy

 Legislation

 Ethical principles.

3. What 'categories' of skills do nurses require to deliver care?

3. Assessment

 Comfort/caring

 Clinical skills

 Communicating and interacting with patients

 Health and Safety

 Organisational skills

 Personal and professional development.

Chapter 2

1. What is different about our approach to skill development?

1. It includes patient factors, the clinical context and the student's learning needs.

2. Why do we need to alter the way we carry out skills?

2. To deliver care that is holistic and individualised, therefore tailored to patient needs

 To respond to changing different clinical situations

 To respond to changes in the patient's condition.

3. Why is it important for nurses to use reflection?

3. To make sense of complex situations, by identifying and exploring the issues, identifying the underpinning theory and suggesting other approaches to similar situations.

4. What 'thinking skills' do nurses use to make sense of patient care needs?

4. Problem-solving

 Critical thinking

 Decision-making.

5. How will you identify what helps *you* learn effectively?

5. Using a tool such as Kolb's Learning Style Inventory to identify what kind of a learner you are and what learning strategies are most effective for your learning style.

 Linking this information to learning environments such as university and clinical placements.

Chapter 3

1. List the six key concepts that are the foundation for all clinical skills delivery.

1. Assessment, communication, risk management, professional judgement and decision-making, risk management, managing uncertainty.

2. What term do we use to describe these six key concepts?

2. Enablers.

3. There are three main ways of collecting assessment data identified in this chapter – what are they?

3. Measuring, observing and interviewing.

4. How does the biomedical model of care differ from the psychosocial one?

4. The psychosocial model of care gives as much consideration to patients' psychological and social wellbeing as it does to their physical wellbeing.

5. What is the challenge of knowing your attitudes and prejudices?

5. You may have to change your attitudes and alter your prejudices. This can be a long and difficult process, as first you have to recognise the need to change and then you have to equip yourself with the motivation to change.

Answers to case study – Shonagh Devine

● **Shonagh is giving you mixed messages. How could you clarify how she is feeling?**

Sit with Shonagh for a while; use touch if you are sure that that will be acceptable to her. Explore her feelings more fully by reflecting back what she has said to you. You could say something like 'I do understand that you want to go home, but tell me more about how you think you will feel when you do get home.' This will give her the opportunity to talk about how she feels. If this is not successful, you could take the approach that she looks tearful/upset and explore her feelings from there.

● **Given the information above, what might be the reasons for Shonagh's ambivalence about having an ileostomy?**

Personal: She feels exhausted all the time; this could be in part due to anaemia and dehydration. The feelings of exhaustion are quite likely to be compounded by depression. Living with a chronic debilitating illness that impacts markedly on a

person's lifestyle often makes them feel as though they have little control over their lives and consequently this diminishes how they feel about themselves and how they can maintain control over their lives. Shonagh may therefore be unable to make any decisions, even very important ones.

Altered body image: If Shonagh's self-esteem is low it is likely that she has a poor body image as well. If this is the case, she may also feel that with an ileostomy she will lose her appeal as a woman and a sexual being. She may think that it will make her unattractive and unfeminine. She may feel that if she has an ileostomy she will have to wear clothes that she wouldn't normally wear to ensure that her stoma stays hidden from view.

Lifestyle: Shonagh may have a number of concerns about having an ileostomy:

– Will it affect the relationship she has with her children?

– Will it affect her future fertility?

– How will she dispose of the stoma equipment discreetly when she's at home or on holiday?

– Will she be able to continue to work as a nurse?

– Will her activities and hobbies be curtailed by having a stoma?

● **What is the most likely cause of her contusions?**

It's possible that Shonagh is suffering domestic violence. Her husband will also have gone through a variety of feelings and emotions during this difficult time for the family. He is probably very worried about his wife's condition and her long-term future. He could feel very angry at what is happening to him, his wife, his children and the impact that all of this is having on his job. He is also impotent in all of this; he can't suffer instead of his wife, he can't do anything directly to ease her condition, he just has to be there. Friends and family could be so focused on helping and supporting Shonagh, Tim and Amy that Dan has been forgotten about. He has a highly stressful job and it is possible that they may have financial difficulties. While none of this justifies Dan's behaviour in any way, it does recognise why he is using inappropriate behaviour to express his feelings. If Shonagh is suffering domestic violence then appropriate help and support must be made available to her, if she agrees.

● **Shonagh has confided information to the dietitian. If you were the dietitian would you make this information available to the rest of**

the multidisciplinary team without Shonagh's consent?

It is important that information given to any health professional is kept confidential. However, if the dietitian feels that it is necessary to share such information with the rest of the multidisciplinary team to improve Shonagh's care then he/she must discuss this with Shonagh and gain permission to do so. Sharing information without Shonagh's permission is a breach of confidentiality. However, the dietitian does have a duty of care and he/she will need to balance this against the need for confidentiality.

Chapter 4

1. **What are the component parts of the skills template?**
1. What is it?

   Why do it?

   Knowledge underpinning practice

   How to do it

   Reflection on action

   References and further reading.

2. **What are the roots of the MASC model?**
2. Patient

   Personal

   Professional

   Context

   Evidence.

3. **What are the enablers in the MASC model?**
3. Assessment

   Communication

   Risk management

   Professional judgement and decision-making

   Record-keeping

   Managing uncertainty.

4. **How do the template, roots and enablers in the MASC model relate to each other?**
4. The roots of the tree are representative knowledge and understanding that will influence your behaviour and thinking. The skills template, which is represented as the trunk of the tree, provides the what, why and how of skills delivery and encourages the use of reflective and evidence-based practice. The enablers are fundamental skills that underpin *all* care and are required for development and sustainability of skills. They equate to the food and water required by the tree.

Chapter 5

1. **List six characteristics of teams.**
1. Teams have shared goals

   Team members are mutually accountable for the work they carry out

   Teams can be formal or informal

   Teams can be permanent or temporary

   Some teams are made up of a variety of professionals, i.e. they are multidisciplinary

   Teams have their own culture.

2. **Why is discharge planning a major issue in health care?**
2. An increase in day case surgery, coupled with higher bed occupancy, results in patients being sent home more quickly than they would have been in the past.

3. **Is your functional role the same as your team role?**
3. Not always. Your functional role might be Staff Nurse, whereas your team role is co-ordinator (Belbin 1993). Belbin suggested that there were nine team roles, based on personality traits, group behaviour and performance within the team.

Chapter 6

1. **Where can you find policy documents?**
1. You will find a variety of policy documents at www.dh.gov.uk/PolicyAndGuidance/fs/en.

2. **How might you summarise the government's modernisation agenda?**
2. a. The NHS has to be redesigned around the needs of the patient, who may be an expert in their own care.

   b. There needs to be more, better paid staff, using new ways of working to deliver this service, with a clear career structure.

3. How would you identify the skills and knowledge associated with your role?

3. Use the MASC model and access the Knowledge and Skills Framework (Department of Health 2003)

4. How would you define lifelong learning?

4. According to the Nursing and Midwifery Council (*Supporting Nurses and Midwives Through Life Long Learning*, 2002, p. 3), lifelong learning is 'more than simply keeping up to date. It requires an enquiring approach to the practice of nursing and midwifery, as well as issues which impact on that practice'.

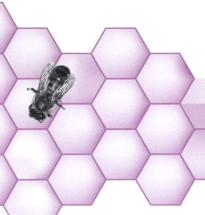

Appendix B

The template and the model

Skills for practice: administration of medicines using a medicines trolley

What is it?

Administration of prescribed medication to an identified patient.

Why do it?

To cure the patient and restore health. When this is not possible medication may be used to relieve symptoms. Some medicines are prescribed as replacement therapies, when the body is unable to produce a particular substance, for example a hormone, in sufficient quantities.

The medicine is therefore prescribed in a dose that is safe for the patient but will be effective, in other words: 'to achieve a certain, predicted effect within the body' (Dewar 2000, p. 14).

Knowledge underpinning practice

- Nursing and Midwifery Council (2002) *Guidelines for the Administration of Medicines*
- How the medicine acts, its normal dose, side-effects, precautions and contraindications
- Knowledge of the patient, their previous medicine history, e.g. allergies and their care plan
- What constitutes a correct prescription
- Dosage, route and timing of administration and drug interactions related to the individual patient (Nursing and Midwifery Council 2002)
- Drug legislation
- NMC (2002) Code of conduct
- Local drug policies
- SI units and calculations
- Related anatomy and physiology
- Safe storage and ordering of medicines and disposal of unwanted medicines
- Hand-washing
- Issues such as compliance, tolerance and dependence, covert administration

- Branch-related issues, e.g. child development, ageing, the Mental Health Act, empowerment and consent.

How to do it?

- Prepare medicines trolley, current oral medicines, appropriate equipment such as spoons, BNF, water, making sure trolley is clean and is able to be secured if necessary
- Consider patient factors such as: identity, allergies and consent
- Check that the prescription is clear and valid
- Check that the dose has not already been administered – this includes regular, as required and once-only prescription charts
- Check any special observations or requirements relating to the medication (Nicol *et al.* 2004)
- Select the medicine, confirming dose, route, frequency, form and expiry date, and dispense in to appropriate measure/cup, calculating the dose where appropriate
- Confirm own knowledge of the medication, such as action, normal dosage, route, interactions and side-effects
- Confirm the identity of the patient verbally, checking the identity bracelet with the prescription sheet (Foster and Hilton 2004)
- Administer the medicine to the patient, ensuring that the patient takes it. Consider the patient's position and ability to comply, and the need to provide a drink
- Reinforce the need for the medication and check the patient's understanding of the medication plan
- Record the administration, or reason for not administering, such as refusal by the patient or other factors such as nausea
- Leave the patient comfortable.

Reflection on action: points to consider

- What part of the action did I do well?
- How could I improve?
- What background knowledge do I need?
- Is there any research related to this activity?

References

Dewar, K. (2000) Introduction to pharmacology. In: Prosser, S., Worster, B., Dewar, K. *et al.* (2000) *Applied Pharmacology: An introduction to pathophysiology and drug management for nurses and healthcare professionals*. Mosby, St Louis, MO.

Foster, J. and Hilton, P.A. (2004) *Fundamental Nursing Skills*. Whurr Publishers, London.

Nicol, M., Bavin, C., Bedford-Turner, S. *et al.* (2004) *Essential Nursing Skills*. Mosby, London.

Nursing and Midwifery Council (2002) *Guidelines for the Administration of Medicines*. Nursing and Midwifery Council, London.

Skills for Practice

What is it?

Why do it?

How to do it

Reflection on action: points to consider

References

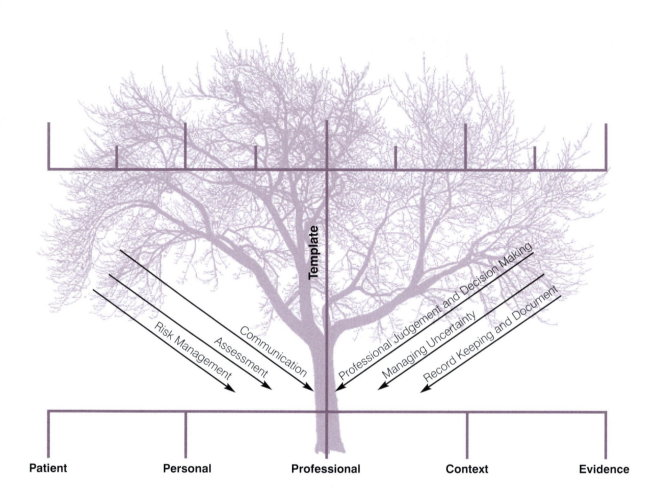

Template

Risk Management

Assessment

Communication

Professional Judgement and Decision Making

Managing Uncertainty

Record Keeping and Document

Patient   **Personal**   **Professional**   **Context**   **Evidence**

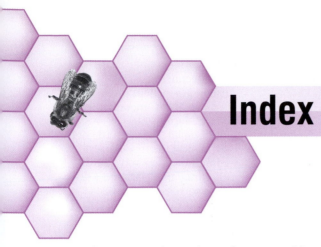

Index

Page reference in italics indicate figures or tables